Weight Loss Lunar Magic

Let the Cycles of the Moon help you lose weight

Julie Ann McBeth

"All the world is made of faith and trust, and pixie dust,"

Peter Pan – JM Barrie

Your horoscope will never be a substitute for eating well and you cannot blame the stars for your weight. You can, however, use the universal cycles, particularly that of the Moon, to assist you with your weight loss.

Copyright

First Printing 2015

Cosmic Imprint P/L

Port Melbourne

Vic, Australia 3207

Illustrations by John Zurbo

ISBN: 978-1-326-51985-8

Table of Contents

Chapter 8 – Choosing the Program for your Horoscope Sign...**104**

Chapter 9 - Now for the Magic! **115**

Chapter 10 – Ready for the Weight Loss Ceremony **122**

Preface

I know that many of you have come across this book because you have tried so many times to lose weight and it has not worked. I understand and have been there too – so I set about to use the skills I have to help you use the cosmic cycles so that your weight loss may be simple, steady and without too much struggle.

Time is of the essence – how many times have you heard that? All it really means is that this moment in time is unlike any other.

In 2008 I was filming a television show and I looked at myself with horror! I knew the camera put on a few pounds but I had no idea I was that overweight. The television show was based on my study of the cosmos – my journey with astrology.

I was giving so many people advice about different topics and doing lots of personal consultations that were really helping people with their problems.

So I looked at myself and thought – What if I could use astrology to help me lose weight? It seemed simple enough.

Last year my sister had her second baby and had gained 30 kilos. I looked at her horoscope and gave her the information that I am now giving you. She has lost 20 kilos and after the Christmas festivities intends to lose the final 15 kilos forever using the same techniques.

Many of us are sick of the different diet fads. We have tried them all and they may work for a while but sooner or later the weight creeps back on.

This book is designed to help you understand your own horoscope – the three key points – your Sun, Moon and Ascendant sign. Then we set a date when the Moon is in its "waxing" phase so that we are going with the cosmic energy flow and not against it. Then we lock in a date and time that will help you stick to your diet plan without any of the emotional fuss.

To get the dates that you need, make sure you follow me on social media or on my website – www.starsandthecity.com

Good luck – May the Cosmic Energy Tide be with you.

Chapter 1 – Cosmic Cycles and Weight Loss

As a Gemini, from the moment I was born, I was asking questions – I probably drove my parents crazy. As I moved through primary and secondary school I could see that books could give me the answers -so I read everything!

But I got to the end of my university education and still did not have the answers I needed. What am I going to be?

I got a good job as a financial journalist, pretty soon I was thinking my life was on track, but it wasn't. So much was missing.

During one phase, I locked myself away for weeks reading books as I struggling to know what to do next. There was one in particular – *How to Cast your own Horoscope* – that I found intriguing.

As a financial journalist I had wandered in one day to find a senior colleague pouring over these pages of hand drawn illustrations – circles with strange squiggles inside them.

Of course I asked: "What's that?"

He said: "They are my astrology charts"

Me: "That's crazy isn't it?"

Him: "Ahhh, no. Why don't I do a reading for you and you can judge for yourself?"

So he did and I became fascinated. How could he know all of this information just from my birth details?

I understand now that this was a very good way to deal with a Gemini who has a big Taurus stellium, (four planets in the same sign) in her first house. I need to experience something – to touch and feel it and make sure it works in a *practical* sense.

Many years later I'm still asking questions and learning about the celestial spheres because it really doesn't make sense. But that is its frustration and its beauty.

From the position of skeptic I slowly started my journey down a very winding road. Up hills, crossing rivers, throwing it all out and starting again (yes traditional astrology) until one day I stopped.

I thought – I am now an astrologer. I can do this. This is who I am. And if the world thinks that I am crazy then it is up to me to show people that it is not.

That it is so profound and so amazing that it leads me to know without question that we are not alone. We are part of a much bigger cosmos. A universe that is so large, wondrous and mysterious that I have no capacity to understand it – so I still have questions – I just don't expect to have all the answers anymore.

I know I can use astrology to help other people find answers. So this is what I love to do.

My own weight loss journey

As a child I was skinny. So skinny that I spent many days in hospital and my parents had to monitor and help me to eat. I had absolutely no interest in food. Until one day I tried pizza…and then a year or so later Chinese food.

So it turns out that I had no interest in my mother's cooking which was the 1970s classic meat, three vegetables and the occasional casserole or roast dinner. Lunch was always sandwiches. Snacks were always fruit with the occasional biscuit and very infrequently a large bag of potato chips shared between the five or six of us.

When I think about it now, it was good healthy food. We always had fruit in a bowl on the kitchen bench. Meals were smaller and the evening meal was always followed by dessert which was usually ice-cream and some sort of tinned fruit or jelly or something that was very old fashioned like bread and butter pudding or sago (who even eats that now!).

Then the hormones kicked in. Every female reading this will know that this pretty much changes the way you look, feel, eat and react to things and in my case I went "puffy". I now understand this, but at the time I was just embarrassed and puzzled as to why my body was changing so much while others were not.

And that is one of the keys to body image, weight loss and healthy weight management – do not compare your body to others! Your body is different for a myriad of different reasons.

So through adolescence and into my 20s I had a body that I had no connection to – I didn't feel it at all. I had no idea what to eat or when to exercise or how much I should be doing so I just meandered along hoping for the best. I must say that due to my good genetic makeup and other factors (such as astrological influences) I managed to look ok but I was not what you call a stunning beauty.

Then when I moved from my home in Melbourne to work in Sydney I suddenly gained weight as I was away from home for the first time and I ate way too much takeaway food. (Aries and Gemini are prone to do this because they are running around crazy and often don't have time to cook!) I was so unhappy and I gained about 10kg (25 pounds).

I became interested in astrology in the late 1980s and in 1992 did my first course where I learned all about the planets and the signs. It was then I realised how lucky I was – my chart is a minefield of contradictions when it comes to my appearance.

I am a Gemini which is a good sign to have if you are looking for clues about body size/weight. Geminis generally run on nervous energy and can be very thin (think Angelina Jolie) as when they get too stressed they often find it difficult to eat. Their mind is always racing and there is too much to do in a day so that food becomes very unimportant (which was like me as a young child).

However, I have the Moon, Jupiter, Mars and Mercury all in the sign of Taurus and mostly in the first house. Now Taurus loves food – fatty, fried (um, like pizza and Chinese food OK?). And Taurus does not really like to exercise – it is like a big bull sitting in a field under a tree, not much action until they get angry then they charge (more about that later).

With this group of planets in the sign of Taurus (which is called a stellium) in my first house which looks after your body and appearance this could have been a big problem except that I was lucky enough to be born with late Aries rising (another indicator that you could be slim).

So I have two slim factors (Gemini and Aries) which kind of cancel out the weighty factors (Taurus stellium) but there is still an underlying tendency for weight gain if I don't keep it under control.

Later in this book we will look at your signs and see what this means for you! (I bet you can't wait and have already had a peek? Lol!)

When you are younger...

The first time I really tried to lose weight was in the 1980s in Sydney. I realise now that I was eating way too much. I would eat a huge bowl of pasta for lunch and later have another huge meal for dinner.

My portion control and understanding of calories/KJ counting was way off the mark. I didn't even realise how much sugar was in soft drinks as I had always had them as a child.

So I purchased a book – The Diet Principal by Dallas star Victoria Principal. (OK so I was a fan of the show and who didn't want to look like Pam Ewing?)

Her Bikini diet consisted of eating lots of dry toast, steamed vegetables, chicken, tuna, prune juice, and slices of turkey.

In the 1980s in Australia, turkey and prune juice was not readily available. After a day of trying to eat apples and vegetables I nearly fainted.

I also thought I should do some exercise and purchased a few aerobics videos (yes real VHS videos folks) featuring Jane Fonda and Denise Austin.

Jane Fonda was hard. She would say – feel the burn!! I could feel it alright – and collapsed on the floor after the first 20 minutes.

Denise Austin was pretty reasonable though. Her tape was pretty basic but didn't knock me out and she had lower impact options for beginners. She was very caring and enthusiastic – she would say: "Come on I know you can do it! Just a few more!"

After a few days of this I thought – how about I just try and vary my own diet so that I eat less and I will try to work my way up to doing Denise Austin a couple of times a week. I will also walk to work rather than catch the bus.

Cleverly (if I do say so myself) I never purchased a set of scales. Instead I went to the local department store and tried on a pair of size 10 (Australian which in those days was about a 6 US) Levi jeans. I had no hope of doing them up. I could barely pull them over my butt!

Every Friday I would go to the store and try on the jeans. I think it took me a couple of months to fit in to them before I finally made a purchase! They looked great! I received plenty of flattering comments. Guys were asking me out on dates. It was a good time.

Over the years I pretty much stuck to this as my weigh went up and down. Denise Austin carried me in to the next century (when finally had to toss out all my old VHS videos ☹ I bought it as a DVD ☺).

And then you get a little older…

In my 30s I had lots of ups and downs with weight. I realised that as an emotional eater (1st house Moon conj Jupiter in Taurus opposite Neptune in Scorpio) I eat when I'm happy but I eat more when I'm sad.

In 2008 I first used this technique and my weigh has been very stable since. Things have been difficult since my hormones have dropped with the commencement of menopause. But I am confident that this works - as it has worked for me, members of my family and friends. Now I am so happy that I can share all this information with you!

Message to our younger selves...

What would we all tell our younger selves now? If you are young – listen up! Older people have a thing called "Wisdom". It is not valued at all these days but it is about listening to the people who have gone before you and learning from their mistakes.

A unique prospect these days – but if you are wise you can learn incredible things from people with life experience. So what would I tell my 20 year-old self about all the things I have learned?

That forms the foundation for this book. I know dieting. I sure know astrology by now. And I understand what it takes to loose and gain weight.

You may be saying – Oh come on!! If you went to Jenny Craig of course you lost the weight! So why have I purchased this book thinking that there was magic?

Hands up all of those people who have joined Weight Watchers, Jenny Craig, any other weight loss group, tried any crazy shake diet, paid gym membership etc and didn't lose any weight?

Yep – I thought so. Don't judge until you get to the end. Paying money to any of the above will never guarantee weight loss. But for me Jenny Craig had the three important components to my weight loss success.

1. Give me a strict plan so I don't have to think about food or I will think about it all day!

2. Give me a weekly weigh in – otherwise I will cheat. I will think – Oh that's ok – I will just do better next week. NO! Go for your weigh in. Just Do it.

3. The Jenny C program has great substitutes for my weakness – like crunchy salty snacks and peanut chocolate bars.

4. Some exercise if I want to, but this will boost the weight loss – it is not dependent on it. This is especially true now that I am a poor old menopausal lady. There is no way I am going to boot camp. (No thank you.)

This was my experience. It will probably not be your experience. To find out about your unique situation and solution there are a number of ways you can do this. And the Astrology section will help you find out what your triggers are, what your substitutes can be and what you need to have in place for your own success.

Chapter 2 – What is the right weight for you?

So many women get caught up in being the "perfect" size. In Australia and the UK they want to be a size 8 or 10. In the US, women are wishing to be a size 2 or 0.

I must say the idea of being a 0 – a nothing – does not appeal to me. And if you take a poll among most men – it does not appeal to them either.

But women don't lose weight for men do they? Mostly it's about comparing themselves to other women, which is totally crazy, but fuelled by the media, fashion magazines and the general idea of what makes a perfect woman.

Hollywood also serves up women who are frighteningly thin and we think this is normal.

If you have ever met an actress in real life you would be shocked at how tiny they really are.

But that is their job! They want to look thin for the camera, because the camera adds pounds and kilos.

This is not you! You are a normal healthy man or woman who is enjoying life – why would you hold yourself up to this impossible standard?

Be kind to yourself. Think about yourself as a human being who has lots to do and needs a beautiful healthy body to live a wonderful life.

What body do you need for your life?

Do you have children to look after?

Do you work hard and need lots of energy?

Do you enjoy sport and being active?

All of this adds up to one thing – you are unique. You are special and you are different to anyone else. Astrology shows me this for sure. There are lots of different shapes and sizes out there and everyone needs to look at themselves as the best version of who they can be and want to be.

An ideal weight need not be something like a Body Mass Index (BMI) or any other rule or regulation about how you "should" look. It is a weight that you feel comfortable. It may be your clothes fitting well. It may be that you need to look after young children and you want to be fit and healthy enough to run around after them.

Make sure you are realistic about this. Do not think that you can lose weight and be as thin as you were when you were 18 for example. This may not be possible. What you want it to choose a goal that is realistic for you in your present circumstances - where you would feel happy.

This is where talking to your GP, a dietician or a consultant can be beneficial. Some of you will even have mothers who can tell you exactly what your perfect weight is – sometimes mothers are very wise – they understand you better than you think!

So make your goal attainable. Make it easy for you to maintain and think of your lifestyle and how you want to feel.

It may be easier for you to break down your goal in to a few easy steps. For example if you have 30 kilos to lose – break it down in to three lots of 10 kilos. Lose the first lot – maintain for a while and then go to the next round.

This is your life and there is no hurry to get in to that bikini! You want to be able to get in to your own skin first and love how you feel – just for you – and don't worry about anyone else. This is your journey – make it simple and make it your own!

Before you start your Lunar Magic

Do you want it? If you really want it you have to stop with the excuses and justifications about your current situation.

Be quiet. Find a place in your home where you can sit for a while and think about this seriously.

What would it feel like to be thinner?

What kind of clothes could you wear?

Imagine looking at your before and after photo. Have faith in yourself. And follow your plan – every day!!

With a little help from the universe and some magic moon times – we can do it!

Chapter 3 – Cosmic Energy – What is Astrology?

Astrology is much more than the horoscope columns you read online or in newspapers or magazines. This is what we call Sun Sign columns – where the zodiac is divided in to 12 different signs and you read the corresponding sign based on the day of your birth.

Some people who were born on a day when the Sun changed signs think they are born on the cusp – so they are a mixture of both signs but that is not right! When you cast your own unique horoscope chart it is for the exact time you were born and the sun will be in one sign or the other. It cannot be in both!

Having your own chart done is like having a couture dress made for you – it is not prêt-a-porter (ready to wear)! It fits you like a glove and that is because your body is not the same as everyone else's.

In the same way, your chart is not the same as everyone else, unless you are a time twin and even twins can have different charts because one was born later than the other.

Astrology is a system of ancient knowledge that relates to the study of the movements of celestial bodies (Sun Moon and planets) and interpreting the impact this has on our lives.

Reading the "language of the stars" helps us to explore the impact the action of celestial bodies has upon people, places, and things (such as countries, cities, events etc) and this can give us some great insight into what is happening behind the scenes.

It is not about reading your horoscope column for the day and deciding that you should stay in bed! Or asking someone (like they did in the 1970s) – what's your sign?

A horoscope is an individual chart that is created by an astrologer, based on your specific time of birth (date, time and place). The chart is like a map of the heavens when you were born and astrologers then read that map to help people with their path.

An astrology reading can give help you to understand yourself, your relationships and your work or career. It can also help answer questions that have been bugging you- like "Does he love me?' or "When will the money arrive?"

Most of all, astrology explains why we are individuals. We are not the same. This is why there is no one-stop shop or quick fix for everyone when it comes to our problems.

Weight loss has been my problem but it is no longer even an issue. I have helped others do the same and it has worked. So I thought you may be interested in how your sign deals with food, weight, willpower, exercise, motivation and the elements that make up a healthy body.

It all starts with your individual chart, so go to my website – www.starsandthecity.com and I will send you a copy of your chart if you give me three pieces of information:

1. Your date of Birth

2. Time you were born

3. Place you were born.

This will give you the three most important signs for following the information in this book:

1. Your Sun sign

2. Your Moon sign

3. Your rising sign

With these three pieces of information you can read about those signs and determine your individual weight loss profile.

We then use the moon cycle to help you cast your weight loss spell and let the magic begin!

Chapter 4 – What's the magic all about?

Let's face it – for most people dieting or losing weight is hard. If it were easy everyone would be slim.

It's tough because there is no pill or potion that can help you lose weight. That would be something most of us would love to have – so think about the ramifications of such a pill. We would have to take it for the rest of our lives and you can believe there would be side effects and of course it would be very expensive!

So why have I called this Weight Loss Magic? What kind of magic can help you lose weight?

It's all about knowing some insights into your personality and unique body type and working with the cycles of time. I know and understand astrological cycles, which is different to reading your horoscopes. It's not about forecasting – it's about picking the "time wave" that will help you to flow with the river rather than struggling against the tide.

This timing coupled with a unique understanding of your own personality can help you lose weight (or gain weight if that's your preference) and will help you "stick with it" which is half the battle.

How many times have you been on a "diet" lost weight and then gained it back again once you went "off the diet"?

What I know and understand about timing and waiting for the right time is like waiting for the force to be with you – and when the force is with you – you can achieve anything.

How can Astrology help?

While I am happy to help with some tips and timing, nothing in this book requires you to "believe" in anything. All I hope to do is introduce you to ancient knowledge that has been understood for thousands of years and was used by people in many civilizations for timing of crowning kings, starting wars and reaping crops.

For those people who want to delve deeper in to the astrology side of things – my website will help you.

But if you just want to use this information for weight loss and choosing the day for starting your diet then it's really important to also read some of the practical information that leads up to the magic.

It amazes me that people may know all this stuff but often unless someone spells it out for them they can't apply the information to their own experience.

If you are nodding your head at this stage don't worry – I have lots of practical plans and easy food and exercise ideas that will help you along your path. None of it is strenuous – I hate gyms and after your 20s they are just plain boring, smelly rooms to be in. Of course some people love to exercise, but my guess is that if you have purchased this book you are not one of them!

Simple is key to making any changes in your life a *practice* - something that you do naturally and don't really have to think about it. So I promise this will be simple. There are no recipes with strange ingredients. There are no other things you need to purchase. It's all right here and I will be on hand to guide you through it all.

How to use this book

In the following sections we will go step-by-step through your plan to help you with your weight loss.

You don't have to read the whole book as some parts won't directly relate to you. In that way, you can use it like a reference book.

We will break it down to a few simple things:

1. Who are you? What works best for you? – Astrology

2. Eating plans for your Horoscope Sign – some diet plans and suggestions.

3. Magic – choosing the right moment for success.

I will also help you with your spell (I did promise you magic) and doing a simple ceremony on the night/day before you start your mission.

But for now – let's take the first step - finding out who you are and what makes you tick when it comes to food and exercise.

Chapter 5 – What's your Sign?

*Dictionary - **Astrology is the study of the movements and relative positions of celestial bodies and interpreted as having influence on human affairs.***

OK. That's probably a good place to start.

It's the study of the planetary bodies: Seven traditional - Sun. Moon, Mercury, Mars, Venus, Jupiter, and Saturn.

There are also a few modern additions - Neptune, Uranus and Pluto. Some people also use asteroids (which I don't but that's up to you) and their movements through the sky relative to where we live here on planet earth. We are on this planet right?

This is very important because as Einstein proved – relativity is central to everything in the universe. If we stand on this planet and look up – this is what we see.

The birthplace of Western Astrology is said to be Mesopotamia. It was then introduced to the Greeks in the 4th century BC and was soon embraced and used extensively throughout the Roman Empire and after the fall, spread to the ancient Arab world.

I say Western Astrology because the Chinese have their own system and the Indians have a different system with a different zodiac.

We are talking about information that has been handed down over roughly 4,000 years. Some periods have been better than others. The Renaissance in England for example was a good time.

Throughout history some of the greatest minds who ever lived have used astrology in their work. Others have either studied it or at the very least understood how to utilize it. Plato, Socrates, Copernicus, Sir Isaac Newton, Shakespeare and more recently Nancy Reagan are just some of the people who are known to have understood the value of astrology.

Today – I think it is growing in interest again and the internet has exploded with information and ideas that have not been mainstream so that people have access to astrological information if they choose to learn about it.

Why there are 12 signs

The zodiac signs are 12 divisions of the sky along the Sun's apparent path around the earth known as the ecliptic. Because we are on a spinning planet, from where we stand, the Sun seems to be moving across the sky.

Of course it is the Sun that is stationary not the Earth. But if you think about this too much you just get dizzy. What's important is that this path is divided in to 12 equal parts, each representing a sign of the zodiac. It's not about constellations (so don't get confused with the rubbish that some groups would have you believe – that there are really 13 signs – there are only 12!)

We begin the year at 0 degrees Aries (because this is when the Sun crosses the equator on the ecliptic). The signs each have 30 degrees and run in order from Aries to Taurus, Gemini, Cancer, Leo, Virgo, Libra, Scorpio, Sagittarius, Capricorn, Aquarius, Pisces.

When you say you are a certain sign of the zodiac this really means that you were born during a specific time of the year when the Sun was in one of the degrees of your sign.

Born on the Cusp

How many times have I heard – "But I was born on the cusp so I'm a bit like both signs."

No you're not. You cannot be two signs. Your Sun is either positioned at 29 degrees 59 minutes of one sign or 0 degrees of the next sign. This cusp nonsense was designed when astrology almanacs where first published.

Before that, people would see the local astrologer and find out what their individual horoscope looked like.

In this day of mass media this has translated to magazines, newspapers and websites giving dates for certain signs. Unfortunately the dates change each year. However the publishers don't make adjustments for this situation as it would be too time consuming and take up too much space.

So now you know. Thankfully we can get an astrology chart pretty easily online these days and you can calculate precisely where the planets were at a certain time and place.

My website will have all this information available. Alternatively Astro.com is one of the best places to find out – or you could do something really outrageous and book a time to see your local astrologer! I also have a list of some good ones around the world who are on my website.

What is a Birthday Chart?

A Horoscope or Birthday chart is a snapshot of where the planets were on your Birthday. And like you it is very individual. There are the three things you need to know to get a chart:

1. The date and year you were born

2. The time you were born

3. The place (town) you were born

Yes it makes a difference if you were born in London as opposed to Sydney. It's a whole other hemisphere with a different time zone and the planet is either in night or day at that time.

Below: An ephemeris is used to show the positions of the planets through out the years.

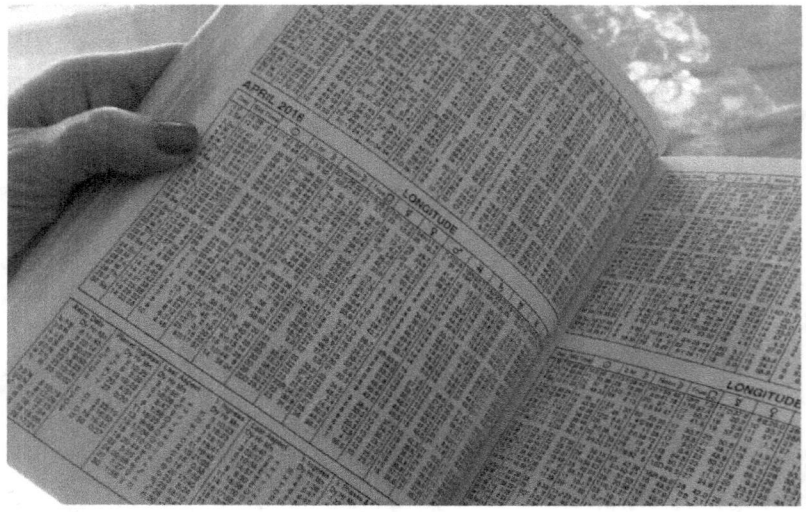

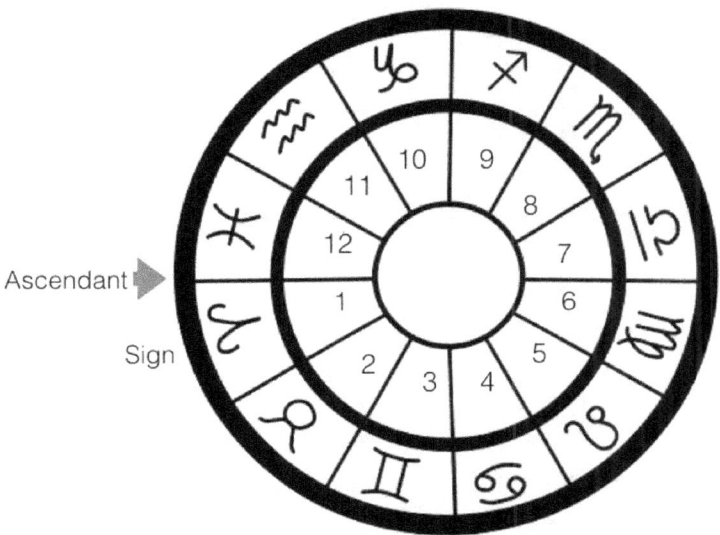

The natal horoscope or birthday chart is divided in to 12 parts called houses. Each represents a certain area of a person's life. There are other types of charts but we will stick to the natal horoscope charts for now.

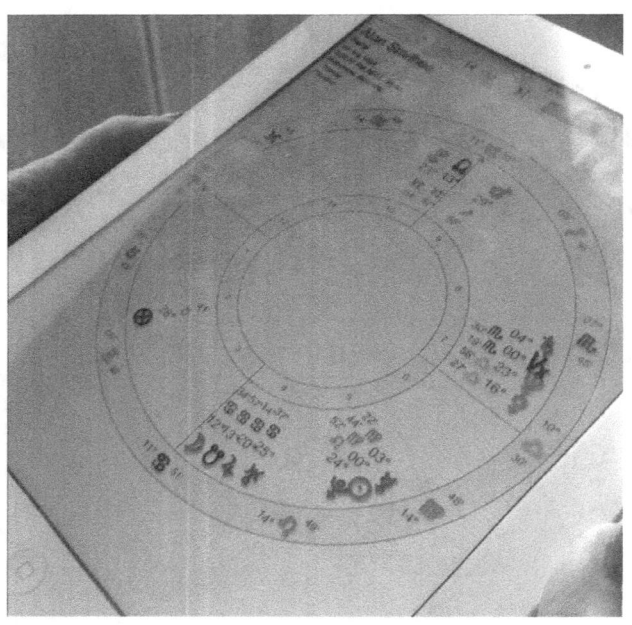

Above: A Birthday Chart (horoscope chart) generated on Astro Gold

As we learned the Sun is found in a different sign during different times of the year. Because the earth spins on its axis giving us 24 hours in a day, as we go through the day each of the signs of the zodiac travel across the Ascendant of the chart giving us what is commonly called – the Rising Sign of the chart. It is the sign of the zodiac that is *rising* when you were born.

This is why it is important to have a birth time. In the USA, most of you will easily find your birth time on your birth certificate. Other countries such as Australia don't require that information so you will have to ask your parents.

What if you can't find your time? All is not lost – don't worry. We can still do a very reliable chart for you based on the Sun – called a solar chart.

This does not give you a rising sign but it will give you a chart that we can work with. So please try as hard as you can to find your time. Go to the hospital records if you can. Sometimes parents publish the time you were born in the newspaper notice.

A solar chart will start with your Sun in the first house and equal houses for the rest of the chart. What we will look at then is the other planets and the moon. The position of the moon can also be difficult to calculate if you do not have a time as the moon moves quickly and could change signs within the date you were born.

If this is the case for you, then read some of the descriptions for the meaning of the moon sign and choose the one that sounds most familiar to you.

The Houses

If you look at your Birthday Chart, you will see it is a circle divided in to 12 slices – a bit like a pizza. And each slice represents a different part of your life.

I like to think of it as the stage or the area of your life that the planets move through. Take a look at your own chart and see where there are lots of planets. You may also have houses where there are no planets. This is OK – so don't worry! For our purposes we are only looking at a few points in the chart.

The Ascendant or the Rising Sign marks the first house and this governs the body and your appearance.

First House – Body, self, appearance, personality, your temperament

Second House – Money, spending habits, financial attitudes, earning potential, assets

Third House – Communications, writing style and ability, study habits, school, travel -short trips, siblings, relatives, neighbours.

Fourth House – Home, father, what supports you in your life, where you live, domestic affairs, what you inherit from your ancestors

Fifth House – Creativity, children, fun and pleasure, love life, dating, hobbies, gambling, social life, any speculative ventures or game of chance.

Sixth House – Everyday life, habits, work (day-to-day not career which is the 10th) pets, and your health.

Seventh House – partnerships, relationships, your rivals and adversaries

Eighth House – Money - joint resources, debt, loans, investments, inheritance, taxes

Ninth House – Religion, spirituality, higher education, overseas travel, publishing, PR, Internet, legal matters, in-laws

Tenth House – career, honours, recognition, promotions, fame, what you are known for, your relationship with your boss and also is the house that indicates your mother,

Eleventh House – Friends, acquaintances, groups, organizations, hopes and wishes

Twelfth House– Things that are hidden from you, secrets, dreams, hidden enemies, your own self sabotage, psychic ability, confinement such as hospitals, prisons etc.

The Signs of the Zodiac

I know you probably know all about your own sign but I thought I would give you a little more information about the signs than the usual stuff because it will make sense to you when you are looking at your weight and how the signs really operate in our lives.

For this we need to break down the signs and understand what makes them tick!

The 12 signs of the zodiac are divided in to two separate groups. The first is four groups of three called Triplicity – this is the quality of the sign. You may know them as elements – fire, earth, air and water.

Triplicity – Fire Earth Air and Water

Fire signs are enthusiastic and energetic.

Earth signs are practical and stable

Air signs are social and intellectual.

Water signs are intuitive and emotional.

Fire – energetic, adventurous, outgoing, enthusiasm, optimistic

Aries

Leo

Sagittarius

Earth – solid, practical, down-to-earth, realistic, determined

Taurus

Virgo

Capricorn

Air – thinkers, intellectual, ideas, communication

Gemini

Libra

Aquarius

Water – emotional, empathy, compassion, psychic, moody

Cancer

Scorpio

Pisces

The signs are also divided into Modality – which is a little more complicated but I have put the meanings here to make it simple for you!

Modality or Quality: Cardinal, Mutable, and Fixed

Cardinal Signs are effective and self starters.

Fixed Signs are focused and determined.

Mutable Signs are flexible and adaptable.

There are also three qualities – cardinal, fixed, mutable

Cardinal – high energy, love of change, self starters

Aries

Cancer

Libra

Capricorn

Fixed – dislike of change, determination, achieve goals, stubborn

Taurus

Leo

Scorpio

Aquarius

Mutable – changeable, go with the flow, adapt,

Gemini

Virgo

Sagittarius

Pisces

So now we can mix and match the signs and get some idea about what each of the signs mean.

Aries – cardinal fire – courage, initiative, impatient, leaders

Taurus – fixed earth – stubborn, determined, lazy, devoted,

Gemini – mutable air – sociable, thinking, communicative, restless, adaptable

Cancer – cardinal water emotional, domestic, nurturing, family oriented, intuitive

Leo – fixed earth – confident, loyal, stubborn, generous, affectionate

Virgo – mutable earth – critical, discriminating, determined but will adapt

Libra – cardinal air - people focus, fair, cooperative, dependent, scattered, flip-flop

Scorpio – fixed water -intense, stubborn, relentless, resilient, distrustful, wary, deep love

Sagittarius – mutable fire – free spirit. indulgent optimistic, sociable, straightforward

Capricorn – cardinal earth – ambitious, cooperative, conservative, pessimistic,

Aquarius – fixed air – independent, aloof, responsible, inventive, intellectual creative

Pisces – mutable water – sensitive, impressionable, self absorbed, impractical, compassion

This is just the basics and we go in to more detail about the signs later.

Masculine and Feminine

The signs of the zodiac are also divided in to masculine and feminine signs. Hang on – what do you mean they are men or women signs? Not at all - this is not a gender attribute and it doesn't mean that because Gemini is a masculine sign that Gemini women are masculine – think Angelina Jolie, Marilyn Monroe – see what I mean!

What this means is that they have qualities that make them more yin and yang.

Masculine signs are diurnal which means they are more active and dry than the feminine signs that are nocturnal and moist. We will get to the meaning of dry and moist – don't worry!

Masculine signs are Aries, Gemini, Leo, Libra, Sagittarius, Aquarius

Feminine Signs are Taurus, Cancer Virgo Scorpio Capricorn Pisces.

Planets are also masculine or feminine.

Masculine planets are the Sun, Mars, Jupiter and Saturn;

Feminine planets are the Moon and Venus

Mercury is common to both genders.

So you can see that the yin, feminine planets and signs are moist and for us that means they are more prone to weight gain.

The masculine signs and planets are dry which means they are not as prone to weight gain. Too much dryness and you may have real trouble trying to gain weight.

It is my background and understanding of astrology that allows me to look at the signs and see how we can utilize this information to help you with your health and fitness goals. It is a combination of the signs, planets and houses that will impact your tendency towards slimness or what I like to call curviness!

Astrology will not say – Oh well you have too much feminine fleshiness in your chart so there is nothing you can do about it.

That is a cop out – there is always something you can do about it. And that is where our free will comes in to the picture.

Our lives are not completely fated. We are able to turn things around and it is by our response and action that we do this!

You just have to be more aware, more organized and have more understanding rather than poking around in the dark and wondering why you gain weight just looking at food while your skinny friend can eat a whole lot of junk food and remain slim.

We all go through different stages in our lives and we can all do something about our lives and change things for the better.

Your astrology chart is like a blueprint. It tells you what you are made of, what you can work with and what your challenges are.

If you can't find a good astrologer or afford a full reading (although I think this is a great idea if you can) then I will break it down for you the best I can so that you can have the information to help you with your goal.

If you have the will, desire, or dream to change your current situation then you can do it, and the magic in this book will help you swim with the celestial river of energy rather than against it.

Chapter 6 – How to Read Your Own Chart

For this part of the book you will need a copy of your horoscope or Birthday chart! You can generate this online at sites like astro.com. There are also some free apps that will give you a copy of your chart.

You will need the following details:

1. The date and year you were born

2. The time you were born

3. The place (town or city) where you were born

If you want a mini reading go to my website and I can have a quick look at it for you and give you some idea of your weight loss capacity and I will give you your key points – your Sun, Moon and Ascendant signs. This is a little bit extra – but it will save you having to work out all the details yourself. You will also get a copy of your chart I can send it to you and you will get a print out that looks like the earlier photo.

You may think: what on earth is this! It looks like a mess but let me tell you, at this point this is your treasure map.

It is your Birthday Chart and it will lead you to information that can help you with weight loss and I can guide you through to make it easy! So don't panic just yet.

As we know from the previous chapter, the circle is divided in to 12 houses and the planets are placed around the chart inside the houses. There are seven main planets that we are interested in and a few outer planets that may be useful.

Your Birthday Chart

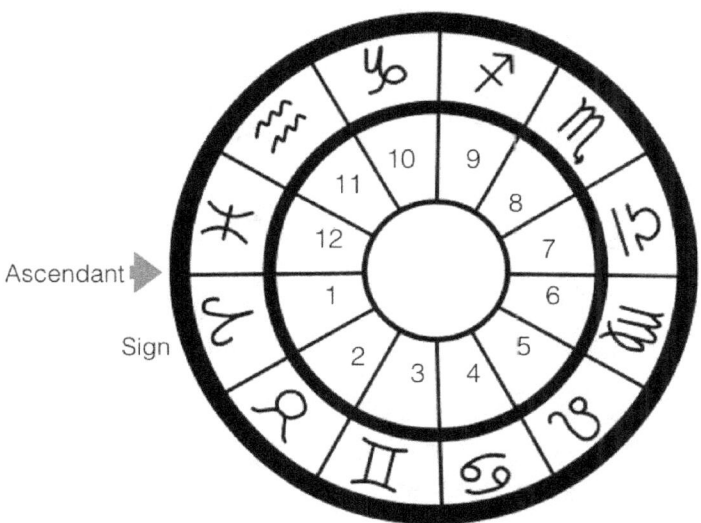

Ascendant ▶

Sign

The circle of your Birthday Chart is based on the position they are in relation to the Earth. Astrologers then interpret the chart and are able to determine characteristics and future events. But for our purposes there are three pieces of information we need to know:

the sign of the Sun,

the sign of the Moon; and

the sign of the Ascendant.

Here is the guide to the signs and the planets:

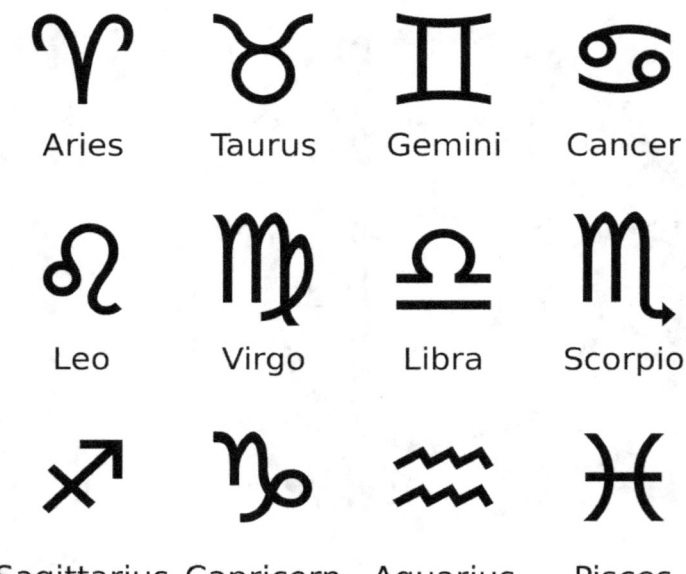

Aries	Taurus	Gemini	Cancer
Leo	Virgo	Libra	Scorpio
Sagittarius	Capricorn	Aquarius	Pisces

What the planets mean

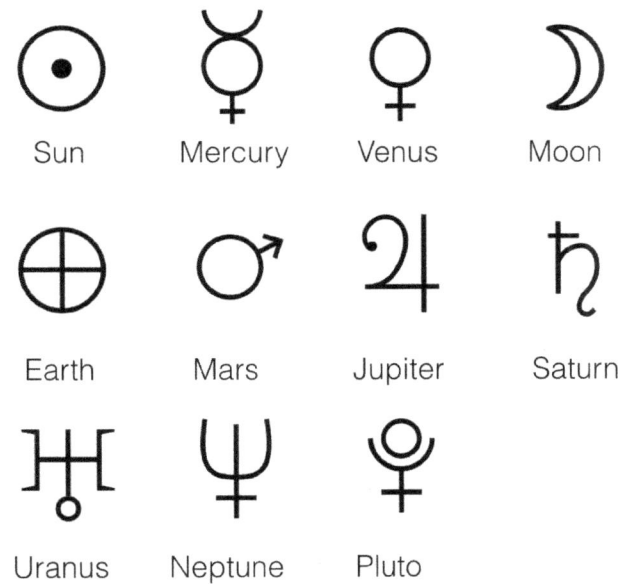

Sun   Mercury   Venus   Moon

Earth   Mars   Jupiter   Saturn

Uranus   Neptune   Pluto

Sun - willpower, ego, who you are, your operating system

Moon - emotional needs, habits, what's important to you for emotional stability.

Mercury – how you think and communicate

Venus – love, money, feminine, what you attract.

Mars – energy, how you get things for yourself, passion and drive, exercise and movement

Jupiter – growth and expansion, luck and fortune, spirituality

Saturn – Structure, discipline, restriction, karma, hard work, time and ageing

The outer or generational planets are:

Uranus – change and freedom

Neptune –spirituality

Pluto – evolution and transformation

Sun Sign

You probably already know what sign the Sun was in on the day of your birth. It is what you say you are – I'm a Gemini or I'm a Leo.

The Sun is not a planet - it is a very big, hot fixed star around which the planets in our solar system revolve!

And as the centre of attention it holds a place of prominence in our lives and our chart. I think this is why most people think their horoscope is their Sun sign. Western astrology is based on the apparent path of the Sun throughout the year as it appears to us from our place on earth.

Have you noticed that the Sun appears to move throughout the year? I know because my windows face south west and during summer the Sun moves around and bursts through my window just enough to make it difficult to watch television, so I have to get up and half close the blind.

We say apparent movement because the Sun is not moving – we are. And based on the fact that Earth is slightly tilted on its axis this gives us the seasons. Remember science classes at school showing the sun crossing the equator at the solstices and moving up to the Tropic of Cancer in the northern hemisphere and then back across the equator.

44

As it does this, it moves through the 12 zodiac signs and when it moves into the cardinal signs – Aries, Cancer, Libra and Capricorn – this marks our four seasons.

This is also the reason you know your Sun sign, as it is the zodiac sign the sun is in when you have your birthday and because it's easy to know – this is how many people understand astrology. But it's not the whole picture...

The Ascendant

To find the Ascendant or Rising Sign of your chart look at the horizontal line that cuts the circle in half. The zodiac sign that is displayed on the left-hand side of your chart underneath this line is the Ascendant or Rising sign.

This is literally where the Sun rises in the chart. When it reaches the top it is generally the middle of the day and when the sun reaches the descendant it generally means it is setting.

So the "TIME" of your birth gives you the circle and the "Houses". This is why it's important to try and find out what time you were born if you can as your Ascendant will give you lots of clues to your body.

Now that you have your own chart calculated, look at the sign on the Ascendant. If we go back to the diagram of the houses you will see that the first house (which is marked by the Ascendant) governs the area of your life related to your body and personality.

The sign on that house (along with any planets here) will also provide extra clues about your body and this can be a real help with determining your weight and your ability to gain and lose weight.

Now go back to the section and read all about that sign. This is the second bit of information that will help us along the path to creating an individual plan for you.

The Moon Sign

The sign of the moon and where it appears in your horoscope chart can also give us some great information about your emotional tendencies. I think it is well known that those of us who are emotional eaters (we get upset and turn to food!) are more prone to be the yoyo kind of dieters.

Take a look at the sign of your moon and which house it is in. For example my moon is in the first house in the sign of Taurus.

Taurus Moons love to be comfortable. And they love the good things in life – good wine, good food but we are the kind of slow when it comes to movement and exercise. So this can be a bad combination if you overindulge in food and don't want to get your ass off the couch to do any exercise then you can be in trouble!

Everyone's Moon sign will affect their emotions and this can be particularly related to your eating and exercise habits.

To find out what it means, go back to the astrological signs and read the sign for your Moon.

The Rest of Your Chart

There are lots of other parts to your horoscope chart that we could look at, but to keep things relatively simple I think it is better to just focus on these three parts – Sun, Ascendant and Moon.

Write them down and look at how they impact on your eating and exercise. For example my list may look like this:

Sun in Gemini – nervous energy, in second house (money spending habits, earning potential) changeable, moody, communication, thinking, too busy to eat, socialable, restless, adaptable

Ascendant in Aries – fast moving, impatient, wants things quickly, good for exercise, may not plan meals, leader, independent,

Moon in Taurus in first house - Body, self, appearance, loves good food, stubborn, determined, lazy, devoted.

So here is a summary: This person is a leader and loves to try new things. They can be moody and changeable at times but stubborn about their body and appearance. If this person is experiencing financial issues or thinking too much about problems there is potential for stress and worry that will lead to emotional eating.

They would need to:

Get some help with planning meals for the week

Do it on their own (independent) but could benefit from speaking with someone on a regular basis about their food and exercise.

Understand that change is necessary to impact on appearance

Probably won't have problems sticking with something if it makes logical sense to them.

Like to exercise but will probably need to do something simple but repetitive – like walking. Will not likely enjoy group exercise (independent)

So now you have looked at your own chart and have got some good insight about your eating and exercise habits we now know what is individual to you and can look for a diet and exercise program that will suit you.

Chapter 7 - The Signs of the Zodiac

In this section I will take you through the 12 signs of the Zodiac. If you are armed with your sun, moon and Ascendant signs you can read all three.

It might be a good idea to write down some notes – because some signs will contradict others and it may be a little confusing.

If you have two of these that are the same then it will be easier to identify your characteristics.

My Sun sign is:

My Moon sign is

My Ascendant sign is

Note any characteristics that are the same.

Note any characteristics that contradict the other sign/s.

Write down the sign's Quality (cardinal, fixed or mutable) and Element (Fire, Earth, Air or Water)

Aries

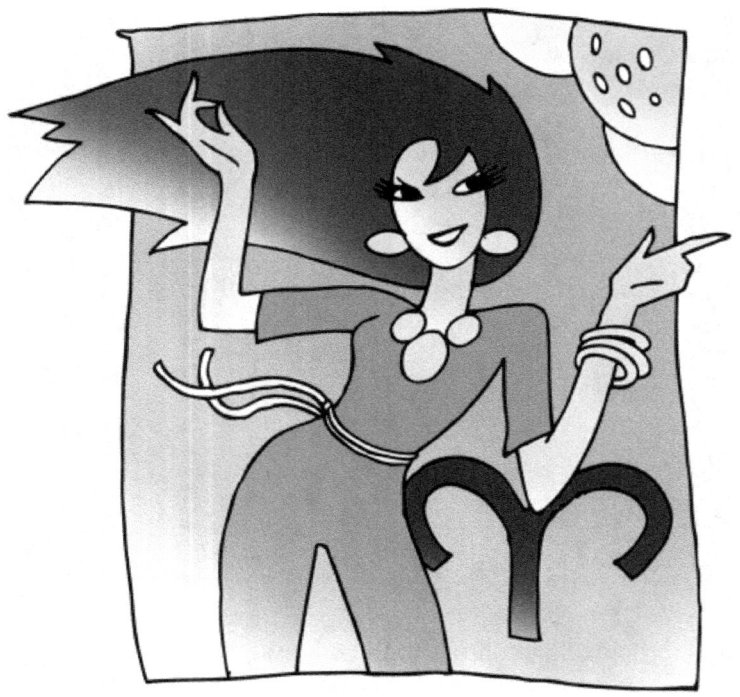

Cardinal, Fire, Masculine

Ruling planet: Mars

Symbol: The Ram

Diet Rating: 7/10

Aries types are the gung ho, go-getters of the zodiac. If you want to start a project or do something that would make you the first in your field, Aries is the best sign to have on your side. They get things done.

Well they may not be there at the finish, but they will start lots of things until they find the one that really grabs their attention and then they can stick to it. They do just about everything fast.

They talk fast, drive fast and walk fast. They want to be the first and they will make it so. They are ruled by Mars which also makes them fearless.

Some may say reckless, but Aries is fast enough on its feet to be able to read the play and know when it's time to make a calculated risk or when it's time to flee!

Brave, pioneer, trail blazing, independent – which is fine but it can get a little lonely. On the flip side are traits like selfishness, self-centredness, or being egotistical or self - obsessed. They are always looking for a fight so stay on their good side and if they look a little angry best for you to move slowly away from them.

Smile – then they won't see you as a threat. They need a worthy opponent and if you smile then maybe you can calm them down. Maybe!

Aries has energy to burn, but this energy can be short-lived. They can Go!Go!Go and then suddenly drop. Their energy is enthusiastic but often not sustainable so they can burn themselves out quickly.

No doubt they are brave – this can often mean they will go where angels fear to tread so don't follow them unless you are sure it's not down some dark alley!

Aries tend to lead with their head and may even have injuries or scars to the head and face.

Often they fail to see the other person's point of view. Me-Me-Me attitude can be overbearing at times.

Impatience is also not your strong suit and you want things to happen quickly – or you get frustrated and this can very quickly lead to you getting angry or just throwing in the towel.

Aries needs to learn when to hold them, when to fold them or just walk away – and of course they often just start something new because that is more exciting!

May start well with lots of enthusiasm but will be very impatient to see results or will just move on to the next project.

Because they are always on the move, it is usually not a sign associated with weight, but other factors may mitigate.

Will probably think it's important to exercise hard and fast at the beginning which could lead to injury and mean they give up.

You like to eat fast and may not take time to savour food or even sit down to for a meal! Getting food on the go seems more your style.

If you are too busy to focus on a diet them this is a good plan for you. The work is done.

You just need to read the whole book. All the chapters – don't just flick through! Make sure you have everything on your checklist before you start. Then let the program fit in around you as just another part of your day.

What Aries needs for success:

Results – you want them fast but deep down you know that it will take weeks. You can't lose it all in one day. Remember – the slower you lose it the longer it will stay off.

You must weigh or measure yourself each week and track your progress.

Set a program and schedule and stick to it.

If you are always too busy to eat – plan meal times. Carry snacks with you.

Know what your substitute foods are and make sure you can get access to them – quickly!

Aries rules the head, hair and eyes and can be prone to headaches. It may be a good idea to drink lots of water (not wine, soft drinks or soda – water!)

Your weakness

Spicy food

Takeaway

Alcohol

Try using spices in your cooking. Put them on salads. Try and increase your fruit and vegetable intake, but chop them up and put them in little containers so that they look like a takeaway meal.

If you must buy takeaway think lots of vegetables, low fat and low sugar. For example don't buy the fried food at Asian restaurants - go for steamed or stir-fried. Best takeaway option for you is Japanese sushi. Wasabi is spicy and will give you the kick you need. Worst is Indian Butter chicken or creamy pasta.

Best Exercise:

Team sports, anything competitive, tennis or squash – something that helps you release energy but where there is someone to beat – you need to win!

Taurus

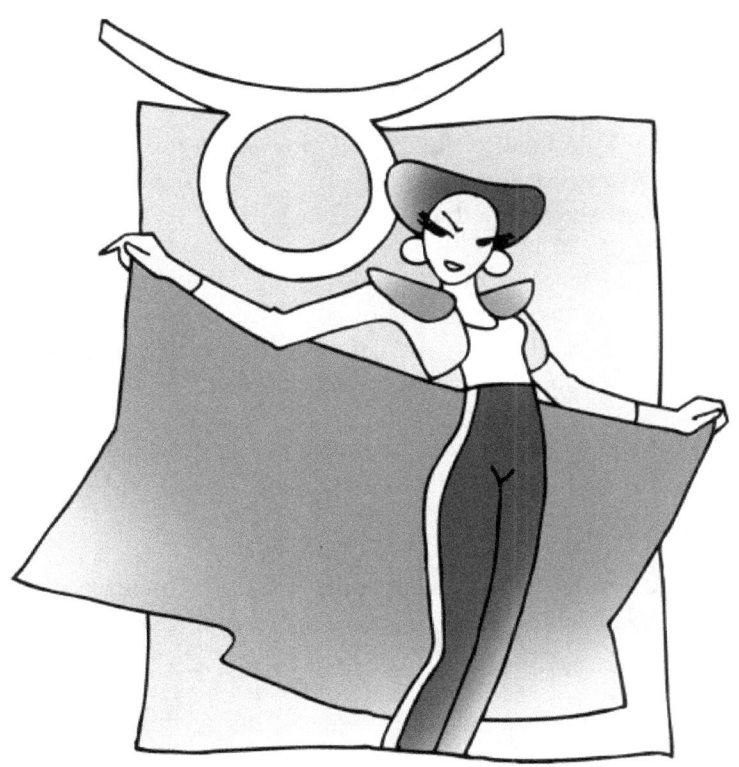

Fixed, Earth, Feminine

Ruling planet: Venus

Symbol: The Bull

Diet Rating: 5/10 (it could go either way!)

Determination is your best attribute for losing weight. Lack of movement though is a tough one for you Taurus as you are a slow moving person and you like your food. Taurus, like the bull, is naturally stocky and unfortunately one of the signs that is more prone to put on weight.

But unlike Aries, which is impatient, Taurus loves a bit of planning and will methodically finish the job. Giving in is never an option. If you do admit defeat then you will have given it a good go before you fly the white flag.

The Taurus motto is I have. So you like your things and money and possessions are important to you. But beauty is another of your finer qualities – you appreciate it in art, clothing and fashion but style must come with comfort.

Taurus is also a sensual sign. So you love food not just for the sake of nutrition and fuel but for the way it tastes, smells and looks.

You love all your creature comforts and sometimes this makes it hard for you to leave your cozy couch – did someone say couch potato?

Stability is important so you must find a way of doing things within your life that will build a strong foundation.

Your weakness is your throat and neck which is also associated with the thyroid gland. This may be something you want to have your doctor check for you.

What Taurus needs for success:

a good diet and exercise plan that can be sustained for a long time.

Something that does not require much movement or strenuous activity

Food that is tasty, looks good and smells good

Rewards for doing a good job

Something that is not too expensive and provides value for money

No pressure – go at your own pace

Set a reasonable, achievable goal

You may not like exercise but you can certainly stay the distance. Your ability to keep going when the going gets tough is your strongest asset. You have the determination to reach your goal. You don't usually like fancy, spicy food.

Your weaknesses:

Food!

Beautiful, rich, fatty food

Sugary food

Fried Food

Wine

Laziness

You don't like change so try and integrate any food substitutes slowly.

Any time you feel deprived you may start acting like a bull – so this is not a good idea.

Instead you need to cut back, rather than cutting out. You can enjoy beautiful healthy meals but they must be with great ingredients and taste sensational.

Perhaps you could start with cutting out any junk food or sweets like chocolate or lollies. Rather than having to have miserable meals – you could just try for lower fat substitutes – like baking rather than frying?

Best Exercise for Taurus:

Gardening, walking, dancing (music is good for Taurus) and aerobics or other exercise set to music. Any exercise you do in nature you would love – so go for a hike in the bush or swim in the ocean. Try to make nature be your inspiration for moving!

Walking is the best for Taurus – but you should walk steadily for a longer time. Try building up from 20 mins gradually until you are around an hour. Intermittent spurts of energy are ok for you but your energy is built for slow and steady not speed!

Gemini

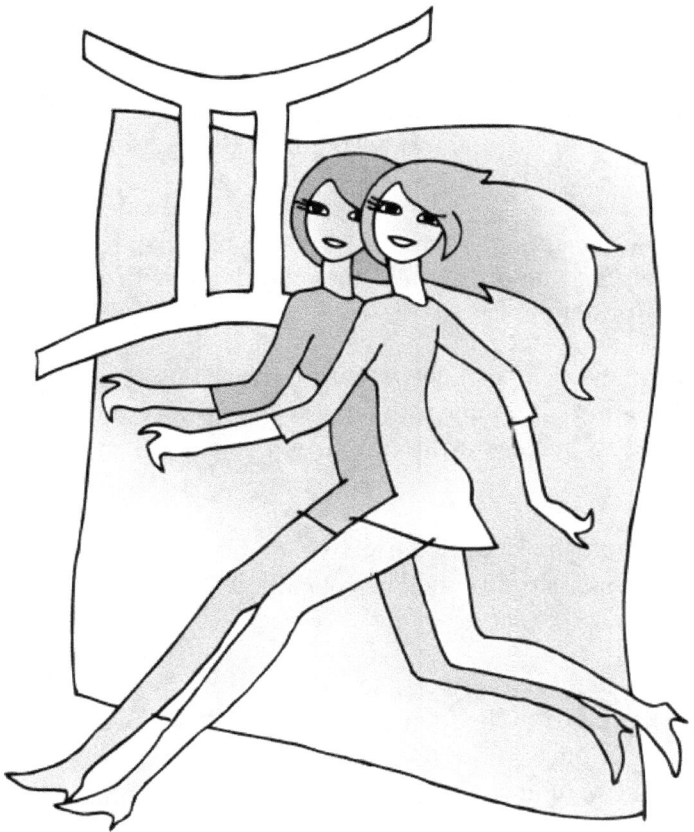

Mutable, Air, Masculine

Ruling planet: Mercury

Symbol: The Twins

Diet Rating: 7/10 – You are generally thin – but gain weight through stress.

Variety is the spice of life for the sign of the Twins. Gemini is a dual sign, giving it a bad wrap sometimes – the two-faced split personality can be one of the major challenges of their life.

Flexible, changeable, and full of information, Gemini needs to be busy and challenged to keep their interest alive. Boredom is to be avoided at all costs!

If you want to know something, Gemini is probably the sign to ask. They are great communicators and their heads are filled with all kinds of information and trivia.

Known for your youthful appearance, wit and style you are a true free spirit. Weight gain is not usually a big issue for you as your nerves tend to keep you jittery and not interested in food.

Alternatively you could be one of those twins whose nerves get the better of them at certain times in your life and you eat to try and calm down!

Sticking to anything can be tricky due to the boredom factor. You love lots of variety in both food and exercise. You love doing lots of things at once – like talking on the phone while you are emailing and watching a TV. (um, I am doing that as I write…)

So juggling is a strong suit but organization and doing things you find boring could be more of a challenge.

Constantly on the go, sitting still is not for you. Yet, exercise can be boring. Going to the same place at the same time doing the same thing is sure to drive you nuts! If you must join a gym then make sure you take a different class each time – mix it up with cardio and weight.

Unlike Taurus, you could never eat the same food every day. So there must be variety added. in to your diet regime.

Use your curiosity and communication skill to hunt down different information.

Get all the info you can about your diet - read the books, calculate the calories. You love getting bits of information from different sources and putting it together in your own way.

Make it a fun game and you could be on track for weight loss success.

The vulnerable parts of your body are your lungs so try to give up smoking if you can. Anything that calms your nerves will be good for weight loss.

Hands and arms are also associated with Gemini so when your hands are busy you are usually happy – think playing the piano, typing, crafts, pottery.

What Gemini needs for success:

A diet and exercise plan with lots of variety.

Something that takes your mind off things – yoga and meditation would be good to throw in the mix.

Try lots of little meals and snacks that you can mix and match.

Something that is not too complicated (or tedious) and you can add your own flair

Set a reasonable, achievable goal and have a buddy or "twin" to help you like a consultant or a friend/family that does it with you or at least is there to talk to and weighs you each week.

Your weaknesses:

Changeability

Nervous energy

Split personality (perhaps one twin doesn't want to be on a diet today?)

Lack of patience – may not plan for meals – take away meals easy option

Too clever – you can outsmart pretty much anyone so consultants have to be strong with you!

Easy to find excuses and you can even persuade yourself not to do this!

Try This:

Think of the fashionable clothes you can wear when you lose weight

Imagine yourself the centre of attention at social gatherings and everyone complimenting you.

Trick your mind with food substitutes – low sugar options

Meditation would be great for you – if you can imagine yourself thinner you can be it as your mind is so strong.

Best exercise for Gemini:

Switch it around – you need variety

Fun – activities that are social and fun like dancing

You love a challenge – so learning something new is good

Social exercise – gyms are fine – so many people to chat to while you are on the treadmill!

Cancer

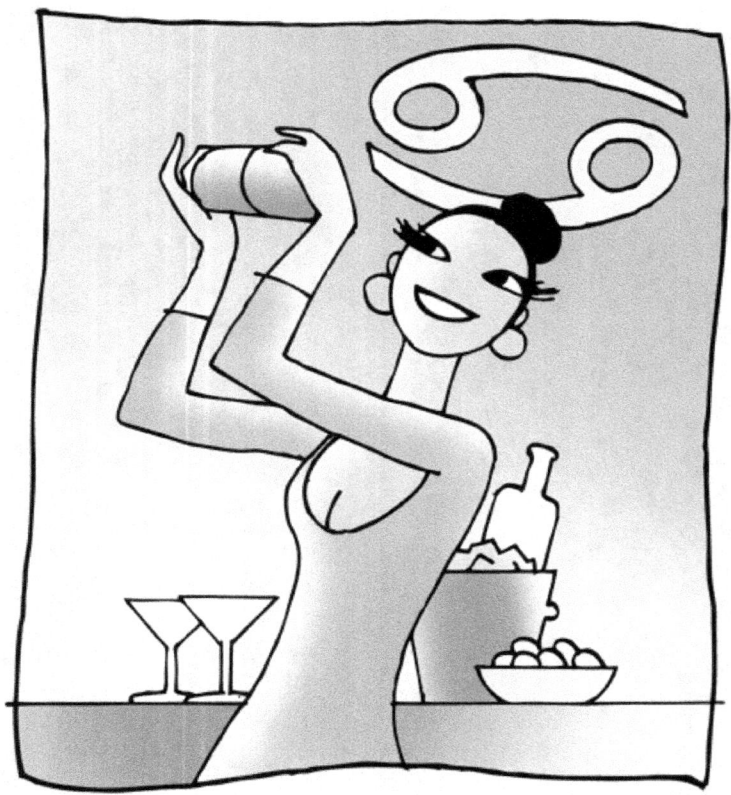

Cardinal, Water, Feminine

Ruling planet: Moon

Symbol: The Crab

Diet Rating: 5/10

What's all this nurturing and motherhood stuff that's often associated with your sign? Cooking, domestic chores, family first - Cancer gets a good wrap as the caring emotional sign of the zodiac.

Well I agree - sometimes you are like this. But other times you can be downright crazy and moody or just absent – hidden away in your shell.

You are ruled by the Moon and are just as changeable.

The moon's cycle is very important to you – so grab your calendar and mark down the full moons for the year. Then you can tell everyone around you that you may be a little crazy around those times and that they need to tread carefully!

The Cancer motto is I feel. That can be tough. And what's better than to soothe the craziness than a nice home cooked meal with all the trimmings.

You love comfort, security, and home. You are usually great cooks and love to entertain at home so you can gather your friends and family around you.

But with all this cooking there is eating right? If you bake the cake you are just as likely to eat the cake!

You are an intuitive sign and people can make you crazy. People at work, people in the shopping centre, people in general. But if you are savvy you know that this too shall pass and you wait a few days and the whole thing blows over.

For Cancer I love the analogy of the United State of America – born on the fourth of July, which is Cancer timing. And what do you associate with the US? Motherhood, apple pie, huge meals, welcoming friendly people who make others feel like they are at home.

You are the Martha Stuart of the zodiac, get the picture? Food is a part of life and showing love and nurturing to yourself and those around you. You attract things to you, maybe its collectables like teapots? Perhaps its cats or could even be people – strays of any kind are welcome.

Cancer is a water sign so you run on emotional energy and if you get emotional you eat. Food from your childhood is what you crave. Just like Mum used to make.

You really do care about people. You hate to see someone upset and will try to fix it. Your heart is in the right place – even if you can be a little moody – your friends and family love you because you care.

Exercise: swimming, water sports, anything you can do at home.

Rules: Breasts and stomach. Your stomach is sensitive when you are stressed so try to keep away from spicy foods and things that upset you, particularly if you are tense or worried.

You have the potential for lots of ups and downs with your diet and exercise plans. Sticking to something is difficult because you get upset and want to throw in the towel.

This is a feminine sign that naturally tends to gain weight, particularly with pregnancy and motherhood (think Jessica Simpson)

It's important for Cancer not to confuse love, home and security with food but this might be a life-long habit to break – passed down through generations!

If you can try to separate your emotions from what you are eating you will be on track to a life time of diet and weight stability.

What Cancer needs for success:

A diet and exercise plan that can help them get over the emotional eating tendency.

Something that does not require much movement or strenuous activity

If you cook for a family try to find a diet book that focuses on healthy family meals

Food that is tasty, looks good and smells good

Something that is not too expensive and provides value for money

No pressure – go at your own pace

Set a reasonable, achievable goal

Get the support of family and friends before you start any diet and fitness regime. You don't usually like fancy, spicy food so make sure it includes variations of your home cooking specials just the lower calorie, lower saturated fat versions.

Try This:

You have your family recipes that have been handed down from your family or that you cook for your family – substitute sugar and saturated fats

Watch the Moon cycle and write down in a journal how you feel at the different stages.

Choose a time when the moon is in signs like Aquarius or Leo. You need a fixed masculine sign that can help you lock down your emotional eating.

Look for low sugar options. Low fat does not mean "no fat" – so look for foods that are high in "good fats" nuts, avocado, low fat cheese.

Exercise at home is good for Cancer. You can do DVDs or apps or work out with family. Take the kids for a walk or go to a playground.

Leo

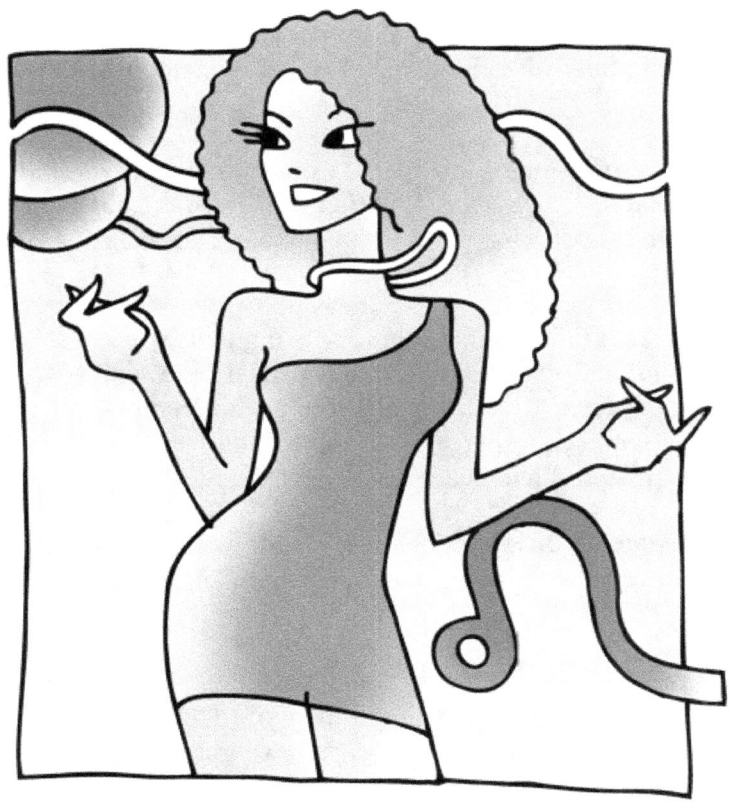

Fixed, Fire, Masculine

Ruling planet: The Sun

Symbol: The Lion

Diet Rating: 7/10

Leo is like the shining brilliant Sun – the earth is revolving around it. As the king of the astrological jungle Leo likes to be treated as such. This means you like to be waited on – to be served and will definitely love the luxuries of life – including food!

Proud sometimes to the point of arrogance, Leo is top dog and likes to be the leader. They need attention and need to be loved – even adored – but what's not to love about a brilliant shining noble Leo?

There is a warmth that radiates through your being that is like the heat of the Sun, and you will share that with people you love - if you are deemed worthy as you are incredibly magnanimous – you will share food, love, fun, money whatever with your nearest and dearest.

But you will not tolerate disloyalty. Ever. Full Stop! Leo is a fixed sign – so once your mind is made up it is unusual for you to budge.

You also love to hold court, entertain and be the centre of attention. If you are loved and understood then you feel all is well with the world and you are unlikely to gain weight.

However, if you feel unloved or unappreciated whether at home or work, then maybe you will reach for the chocolates – a big expensive box with a bow?

Sometimes overweight is just a symptom of your bon vivant lifestyle – the finer things in life and a little too much excess?

Not generally prone to weight gain unless you go overboard with the party lifestyle!

If this is the case then – perhaps you should just cut down a little?

Leo cannot live very long with a bleak lifestyle – stinginess in any form is not your style. You may be better to stick with your usual routine and foods but just cut them in half. Eat on a smaller plate?

If you are having a salad meal then make it a beautiful huge salad with lots of expensive ingredients that you love and serve it on fine bone china with some ice water in a crystal wine glass so that you feel that your lifestyle is being maintained.

If you need an excuse to get off the couch and move, although most of you will do this naturally, appeal to your vanity – do you look good in your clothes or would you like to look a little better?

Social groups and sports such as golf, cricket, bowling and other activities that you can be the life of the part and enjoy some fun will generally appeal to you more than being a lone wolf and sweating it out at the gym.

Gyms may not really be for you do you really want to be in front of a huge group of people not looking your best with your mane perfectly groomed!

That said, look at famous Leo women like Madonna and Jennifer Lopez. For them exercise is about looking good. They have to have fun while they do it and they need people to be watching and commenting on how fabulous they look.

Leo quote – "I've never actually been in a gym – I've filmed in one – does that count?"

JLo – "You got to work out you got to watch what you eat. It's a job – you've got to buckle down."

As a fixed sign – Leo is able to buckle down quite easily once they set their mind on something and if it will give them the attention and comments that they crave!

What Leo needs for success:

A diet and exercise plan that is not too severe – better to just cut back on food rather than try to force yourself on a diet of things you don't like to eat.

Exercise or activity that is fun and social or serves a vanity purpose

You will stick to the plan so make sure your social engagements are under control – so don't try to begin a new regime around the holidays!

Build your partying and social schedule in and find ways around it – like eating a small meal before you go to a function so that you are not starving and eat all the finger food.

You love to add your own creative flair to any regime – so perhaps you can blog about it, take some Selfies and offer advice to others?

Something that looks expensive, regal and luxurious appeals to you – so don't skimp on setting the table, making things look glamorous.

Set a reasonable, achievable goal and go for it Leo – hear you roar!

Try This:

Try to eat what you want but just eat half – you are one of the few signs who could pull this off with your will power alone.

Make your exercise social and fun – join a group activity or bring friends along for a game

Watch the alcohol and food when partying and substitute high calorie cocktails and beer for lower calorie vodka & soda or wine.

Substitute sugar for low calorie sweeteners (you are sweet enough)

Leo rules the heart so perhaps look at a few of the books that have healthy heart diet plans

Your key phrase is I will – in the words of a leader – make it so.

Virgo

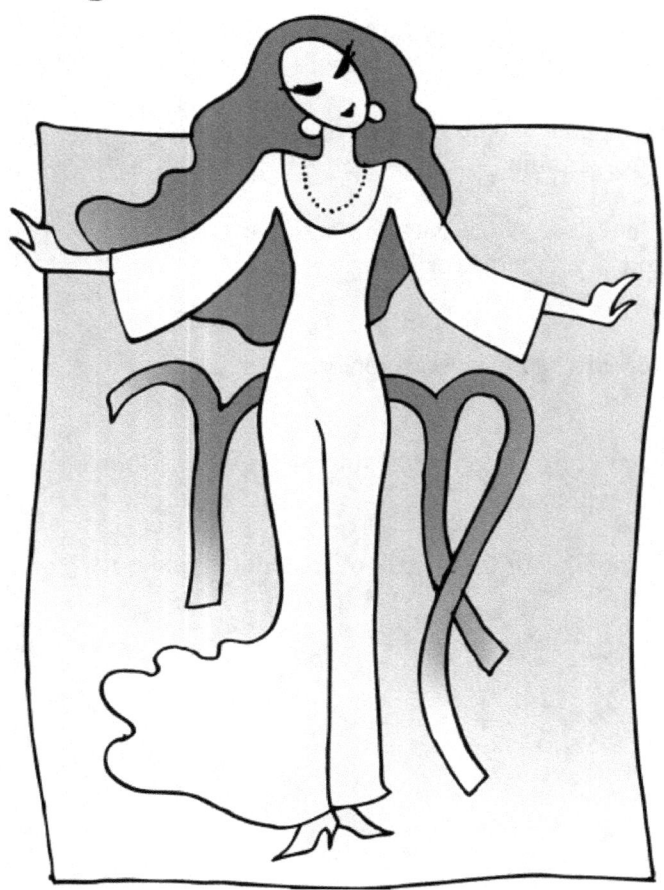

Mutable, Earth, Feminine

Ruling planet: Mercury

Symbol: The Virgin

Diet Rating: 8/10 (not perfect but pretty close!)

Virgo is practical, critical and efficient. You over-think, you over plan and you get a bad wrap for being a neat freak and perfectionist. You also worry about health and hygiene. You are clean.

If Leo is the party then Virgo is cleaning up after the party. You love restoring order and making sure everything is back in its place, then when you feel organized, you can relax.

But Virgo is also a sign of service – you need to feel needed. And sometimes this can be difficult to the people around you who are less organized and who like to just go with the flow. It would be difficult for you to do this – but maybe try it once in a while and you may find it OK. The sky doesn't fall in because you have been less than perfect.

All this organization should mean that your health and diet regime is in check and that you have a list of pills and vitamins that are stored alphabetically in your cupboard so you can find them easily and effortlessly. Maybe you work in a health profession anyway?

Mercury may be the culprit here if you are not. Mercury is the trickster of the planets and it can turn and spin on a dime. This makes you flexible to some extent but worry and nerves effect you.

Unlike Gemini the other mercury ruled sign – your worry is in your stomach, your intestines. You may have a list of food allergies and foods that you cannot digest easily – particularly when you are upset.

What upsets you most is other people's lack of respect to your superhuman efforts to serve them. This can drive you crazy – can't they see what you do and how you have done to the end of the earth to make them happy?

You can also get upset with yourself for being less than perfect – maybe I should have tried harder? Perhaps if I had just stayed at the office for another four hours until midnight then this work would be perfect?

Virgo is the typical workaholic of the zodiac. You love to work making lots of to do lists and checking them twice, or three times or maybe four. You go through every option but when you take it too far you can be paralyzed with fear – so you do nothing.

Your symbol is a Virgin who is holding a sheath of wheat. This is because she has worked hard to harvest it. It doesn't mean you are pure than the driven snow and someone who is taking the moral high road - you are discerning.

Virgo likes to analyze projects and people. At the end of the day, you are intelligent, practical and well organized. In the diet and fitness world – what's not to love about that?

You are able to analyze the problem and you will work hard to achieve your health and fitness routines. To some Virgos their body is their temple. They look after it, and can be very fussy about the foods they will and won't eat. And they will be ultra critical of anyone trying to tell them otherwise!

Think about people who go to diet and exercise extremes cutting out food groups and measuring out everything painstakingly and perfectly and you get an idea of how far you guys can take this diet thing. Very seriously! You do worry a lot however and anything less than perfect may cause you to give up too soon. So you need to make sure the moon is in a fixed sign when you start your program to give you that extra boost.

What Virgo needs for success:

A structured eating plan that can be followed to a "T".

All the rules laid out in detail.

Room in their eating plan for all their food "issues"

Someone who helps them for a change

Be kind to yourself – its weight loss not brain surgery

Try This:

Look at diet plans that work with your food criteria – if you are vegan search for a vegan diet.

Paleo and strict diet regimes may be OK for you

Meditation – take your mind off your worries and visualize your weight loss and how much people will ask you for your opinion and help so they can do the same!

Book in your diet and exercise meetings in your schedule and keep a diary of what you eat

Workaholics sometimes forget to exercise or eat well. So try and book this in to your schedule. If you can make a weekly appointment at the gym with a fitness instructor this usually works well for you as it is just another appointment to check off your list.

Don't worry about doing everything so perfectly.

Look at the long term goal and the path you need to get there. If you fall off the wagon occasionally all is not lost!

Exercise: Think of your health and fitness as a job and try to simply incorporate healthy food and exercise in with your daily routine.

For you, anything that will help with your appearance appeals to you so the key here is not to aim for perfection. Try to do what you can and if you miss a day don't think that it's the end of the world.

Try the simple things like walking or riding a bike and try to relax!

Libra

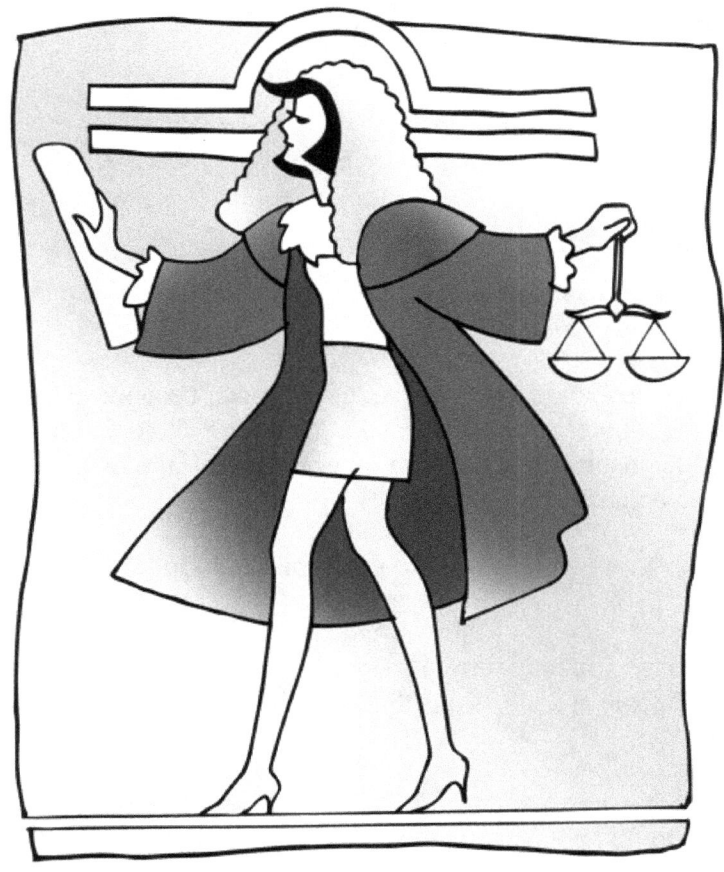

Cardinal, Air, Masculine

Ruling planet: Venus

Symbol: The Scales

Diet rating: 5/10

Librans love beauty, harmony and peace. You dislike arguments and discord and prefer to be nice and friendly – ah perhaps a little too nice and friendly at times just to keep the peace?

Your symbol is the scales – of justice. As an air sign you love to circulate and socialize chatting with people of all types from all backgrounds.

Jewelry, clothing, beautiful objects, art and music are all things that appeal to your senses. So are lollies and candy - sugary sweet delicious candy.

Yet your world is surrounded with decisions. You can become overwhelmed with choices – what if I make the wrong choice? Perhaps I should consult someone? The other person is sure to know what I like better than I do...um no!

If this sounds like you – you may be too gracious and kind for your own good.

When out of balance you may turn to food as a way of seeking revenge against people and situations that you did not stand up to.

You could have, but you would have caused...a scene! God forbid that you should be the person upsetting the crowd.

Sometimes you focus all your attention on others – to your own detriment. You make decisions to please other people.

You follow them or try to get a win-win solution so that everyone is happy – and usually this means that everyone is not happy – least of all you!

When indecision meets self-indulgence – well – Houston! We have a problem and it's going to go straight to your hips.

You need to restore balance. Harmony needs to be your middle name, but not at your expense. Say what you feel and let people know if you are upset about something.

Try something radical like putting yourself first – then when you are happy others will be too.

You are talented and intelligent but may rely too much on pleasing other people. This creates havoc with your diet. (Think Libran yo-yo dieter Kim Kardashian or if you are a little older – Fergie the former Duchess of York who has now turned spokesperson for Weight Watchers – she worked it out!

When all is well then you can stick to a diet and exercise plan – but when you are out of balance it all goes to hell in a hand basket and you reach for the sweetest most calorific foods you can find to console yourself and make everything right again.

Librans enjoy social settings and mingling with people – relationships are important to you. How is your relationship with food?

Good taste and elegance are important to you – so you would love to present yourself in a way that exudes grace and charm. Think Librans Gwyneth Paltrow and Catherine Zeta Jones.

You don't usually enjoy solo activities so pairing up or working within groups is important for them to stay on track and balanced.

You can be a bit lazy at times so you need to choose a moon time where you will stick to your program and gain enthusiasm – the moon in a fixed fire sign like Leo would be good.

What Libra needs for success:

A diet and exercise plan that is not too severe – don't cut out whole groups of foods like carbs – try to aim for balance – a little bit of everything in moderation is ok.

Exercise or activity that is fun and social or serves a vanity purpose

You will stick to the plan so make sure your social engagements are under control.

Build your partying and social schedule in and find ways around it – like eating a small meal before you go to a function so that you are not starving and eat all the finger food.

Share your experiences with others –post selfies on social media, offer advice to others like Gwyneth does on Goop!

Something that looks refined, beautiful and elegant appeals to you – so don't skimp on setting the table, making things look good.

Set a reasonable, achievable goal and go for it.

Try This:

Sugar substitutes are important for you – look for low sugar foods that still taste good.

No sugar diabetic sweets, candy, lollies can also be good snacks.

Treat yourself to the hair salon or spa rather than food as a reward Team up with a partner or someone you trust for advice to help you as you work better with other people and you don't want to let them down.

Scorpio

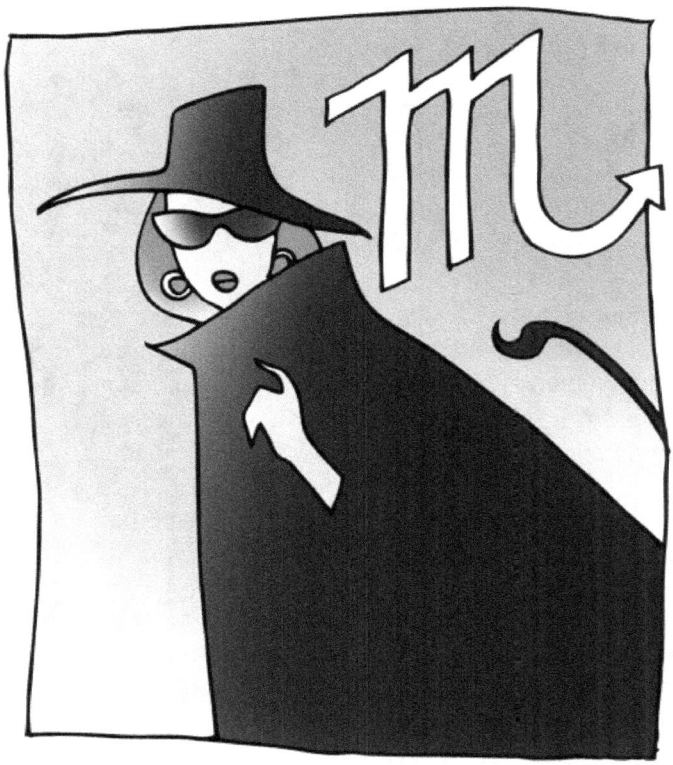

Fixed, Water, Feminine

Ruling Planet: Mars (No you are not ruled by Pluto. Be thankful)

Symbol: The Scorpion

Diet Rating: 8/10

The intensity of Scorpio energy can be overwhelming if you are not used to it. Determination is one of your key strengths – so much so that sometimes it is important to know when to stop as you can be obsessive.

If you apply this intensity to your health and fitness you may be incredibly lean and fit. Mars is your ruling planet and Mars is all about action. But rather than Mars with Aries energy that simply goes for it and charges ahead – Scorpio action is a little more reserved and calculated.

Like your fellow water signs – Cancer and Pisces - you like to feel that your intuition guides, but with Scorpio it's a bit more psychic than intuitive and you need to follow your own advice. Listen to what information comes to you and how you are reacting to people and situations.

You love to drill deep down to the depth of things whether they are issues, tasks situations or relationships. You want to know it all – and you don't take anything on face value.

Relentless pursuits or your goals can be tiring yet you have an innate way of recharging and being able to continue against all odds! People admire you for your endurance

Yours is the sign that deals with all kinds of waste and output. You are not afraid of the underbelly of society or the dark mystical side of topics like death. So a book like this would be fascinating to you on one hand but on the other it may not be deep enough for your mind.

If you need more information there are plenty of ways to research astrology online or book an appointment to see an astrologer – although it could unnerve you to know that someone knows and understands all your secrets…

Endurance, Willpower and a drive to succeed give you the best ways possible to deal with health and fitness issues. Generally speaking Scorpio is a slim sign and you may even have difficulty keeping weight on if you are not careful.

You need to be passionate about food for it to even interest you beyond fuel.

Elimination may be an issue for you as Scorpio rules the colon and bowels make sure there is enough roughage in your diet to ensure you are not constipated.

Passion is the key to your success and as one of the sexy signs of the zodiac you always want to look good in the bedroom.

Secrets are a big issue for you – so if you have an issue with food, diet exercise or anything of that nature you are likely to keep it hidden.

What Scorpio needs for success:

A good diet and exercise plan that can be sustained for a long time.

Food that will keep you going all day is good as you enjoy strenuous activity

Pay off for the work you are doing with any health and fitness regime.

Something that is of interest to you – whatever you can be passionate about will be the best type of activity.

As a water sign water sports may be a good option

Deadlines, pressure any kind of obstacle is good for you as you are determined to overcome adversity

Set a goal that is outside what you think you can achieve and strive for it !!

You may not love exercise but you can certainly stay the distance. Your ability to keep going when the going gets tough is your strongest asset. You have the determination to reach your goal.

Try This:

You don't like change so try and integrate any food substitutes slowly.

If you are a soda drinking fanatic for example, don't change to diet soda and drink it by the gallon. Try and switch to water with some low calorie flavouring or fresh fruit juice infusion.

You love rewards and treats but if your emotions get the better of you do not punish yourself and stop eating.

The flow of your life should be reflected in your diet. Try not to get stuck.

Eat high fibre foods and plenty of fruits and vegetables as these will help with the colon and elimination. You don't want the toxins to build up so drink plenty of water to flush this from your body.

Look for low sugar options but whatever you do leave the fats alone! Low fat does not mean no fat – so look for foods that are high in "good fats" nuts, avocado, low fat cheese.

Scorpio Exercise:

Running and anything that requires energy, muscles and endurance is where you excel. You may love lifting weights but make sure you balance this with cardio work. Remember, too much intensity may not always be a good thing!

But let's face it – the physical exertion you love best is in the bedroom not the gym! A good sex life is very important for Scorpio and it is one area of your life that you need to ensure is flowing well. If for some reason it is not, this could also be detrimental to your body and health.

Sagittarius

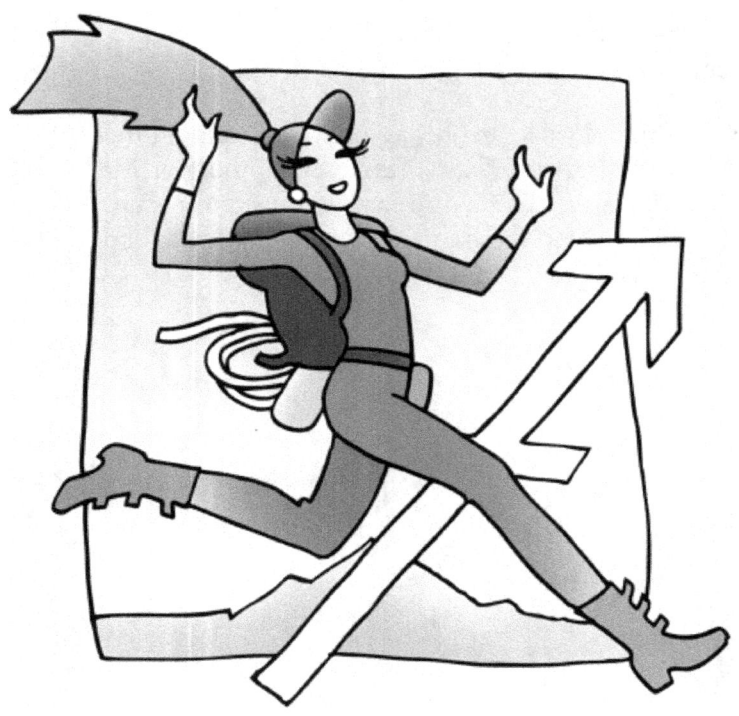

Mutable, Fire, Masculine

Ruling planet: Jupiter

Symbol: The Archer

Diet Rating: Medium to Poor 5/10

Sagittarius rules the hips and thighs and many of you are sighing now at the mere thought. Either they are fabulous like Taylor Swift or not so good like Anna Nicole Smith on a not so good day.

But remember Anna Nicole was once one of the hottest models in the world. Her figure was a reflection of her inner turmoil and that my dear Sagy is the key to it all. You are so optimistic and adventurous that sometimes you don't see the hidden agendas of others.

Your kindness can be taken as gullibility and sometimes people just don't get your "Pollyanna" view of the world. But in the words of Taylor Swift you need to "Shake it off".

If you don't shake off the negativity of others you may turn to food to make you feel better – or worse - drugs and alcohol to restore your positive view of the world.

You are flexible and versatile so it is easy for you to spin around and try to be what people want – but it is your honesty – sometimes to the point of bluntness that can get you in or out of trouble!

I often call Sagittarius energy foot in mouth disease. Sometimes you just say the wrong thing at the wrong time and offend people when you really didn't mean it at all! And you are shocked that they could take offence.

Your other key facet is that you are an information and spiritual guru. You love to travel and explore other cultures and you are not phased by strange ideas or other religious or social situations that may be uncomfortable for others.

You do love sports but you can be the type who loves to watch them from your couch! If this is you, perhaps you loved a type of sport when you were in school and you need to think about taking it up again?

You love to explore and live life to the full but your hips don't lie – what are they like at the moment? How to you want them to look?

As a Sagittarius you have the intelligence to educate yourself about your diet and a fitness regime but it's like you can't be bothered until you really, really, *really* need to – and then it can be too late.

You are optimistic that things will be ok – but sometimes they need to be sorted. Just do it should be your motto!

Sagittarius is ruled by Jupiter – the planet that makes things bigger and this explains your need to live life large. But it can also mean that your love of excess winds up on your body and can take a big wakeup call – like an illness – before you will do anything about it.

What Sagittarius needs for success:

You need a plan. While you are one of the most optimistic signs, failure is an option!

You can easily get caught up in a new adventure and forget about your goal.

Decide what is the biggest motivation for your weight loss? – is it your health?

Get Real – ask people around you who you trust and will be honest Try very hard to be honest with yourself. It's not a failure to ask for help.

Understand that sometimes structure and rules are good for you. You are often accused of just looking at the big picture – which is fine – just make sure you have the details under control too.

Get some help. Seeing someone like a consultant is not failure! Help is good but remember, in the end you need to do this on your own, for yourself. No one can do it for you!

Do you want to wear a smaller size? Do you have a special event where you want to look fantastic?? Think about this for a while. What are the consequences if you don't achieve your weight loss? Will you easily sabotage yourself? Hmmm.

Yes I can see you have lots of excuses. You are now wavering. Maybe you can't. Maybe you are just meant to be cuddly/curvy? Aren't you just like Kim Kardashian? After all doesn't she have curves and millions of fans around the world??

WAKE UP Sag!!!! Kim Kardashian is very petite. She gains a few pounds and looks curvy. But she is probably wearing a US size 6-8 – maybe even a size 4 when she does one of her diets for a magazine photo shoot or special occasion. Yes she is curvy but she is not overweight or obese.

Try this:

Get out and move! You love sport so try something that get's you excited – like archery perhaps?

Nature appeals to you – so hiking in the bush or kayaking down water rapids would be a blast

Channel your enthusiasm in to your weight loss – get a friend excited and share the experience with someone.

Capricorn

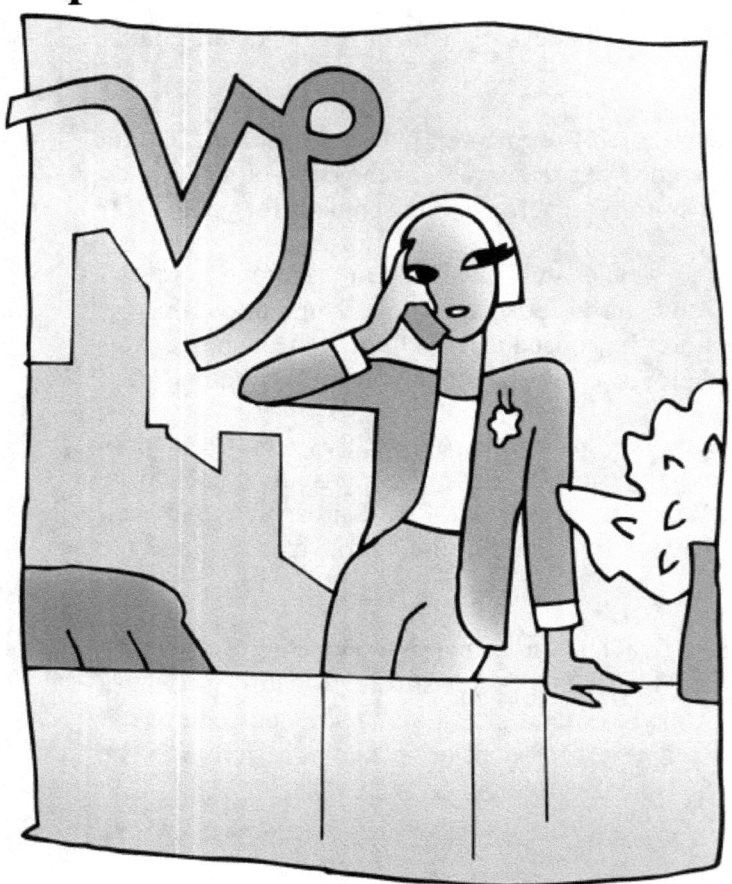

Cardinal, Earth, Feminine

Ruling planet: Saturn

Symbol: The Goat

Diet Rating: 9/10

Ambition meets perseverance! Capricorn can do just about anything it sets its mind to – and that includes loosing weight.

The good news is that you are one of the most naturally thin signs of the zodiac. Ruled by Saturn you are structured enough to be quite diligent at work and you are someone who people can rely upon.

Like the goat that is the symbol for Capricorn, you will slowly but surely make your way up the mountain.

Each time I see those crazy goats on the internet that look like they are suspended in mid-air because they are up on a huge slope that looks impossible I think of Capricorn – for you - anything is possible!

Are you a big time business executive with ambitions to conquer the world? Or a busy mum who likes to organize everyone? You also like to make sure the rules are obeyed and everyone is doing what they need to help?

Yep, thought so. That's you. But sometimes you worry that you need to do more. That the world is such a harsh place and you need to be perfect and follow all the rules and then everything will be ok.

But wait a minute – how come you are overweight? This is wrong. You are slim and too busy for this weight loss shit. How can you fit just one more thing into your schedule?

You are very hard on yourself. See the thing is that you can't stick to a timetable all the time. You can watch your clock – see time ticking away and not enough hours in a day – oh yes you are always on time (unless you are really out of balance – but that's another story...)

And frankly, taking time out for eating is not really your thing. You could make just one more phone call, or write another important tweet or email or just about anything that would put you up the ladder, but…

You could also be one of those people who has always been thin, eating whatever you like and then suddenly, one day in your thirties you think – what's with the weight gain? How did this happen?

If your metabolism has caught up with you it could be baby weight, hormone changes or simply a change of lifestyle – you gained or lost a partner or you moved countries for work and you haven't had time to establish a new routine.

You are hardworking, practical, responsible and at times stingy. All elements that give you a Triple Gold Star weight loss rating!

Self-discipline comes easy for you. And at the end of the day – that's all dieting is about – setting a plan and sticking to it.

It's really important to stop for a minute and be kind to yourself. You can do it – Yes you can!!

What Capricorn needs for success:

Set a reasonable achievable goal with a *deadline* (you love deadlines)

Be practical about your time – are you really going to go to the gym?

Watch your knees and back – don't go out too hard with an exercise program. These are your weak spots – look after your joints (you'll thank me later).

Rather than cut out food groups, reduce your portions (Saturn is all about less so this should be easy)

Count calories, lower your sugar intake, smaller portions and consistency are your goals.

Weigh yourself at least once a week – you need confirmation that things are working.

Learn by doing – you love trial and error and the practical experience it gives you.

If you joined a weight loss club like weight watchers you would be striving to win each week (you love competition!).

Celebrity Capricorns like Kate Moss and Kate Bosworth are easy to spot – tiny and ultra thin but Nigella Lawson (yes the domestic goddess has curves with lots of ambition) and Kirstie Alley (made plenty of cash from her weight loss struggles!) may be more of a surprise.

You worry when you think that people see the chinks in your armor and that they will see you as a failure. Who cares what they think? Any skeletons in your cupboard or any sub conscious stuff that you refuse to deal with needs to be dealt with or the yoyo dieting could be a problem for you. Start with your father and your family and see what you can dig up.

Don't worry – have a think about it and we will deal with it when we get to the magic part.

Aquarius

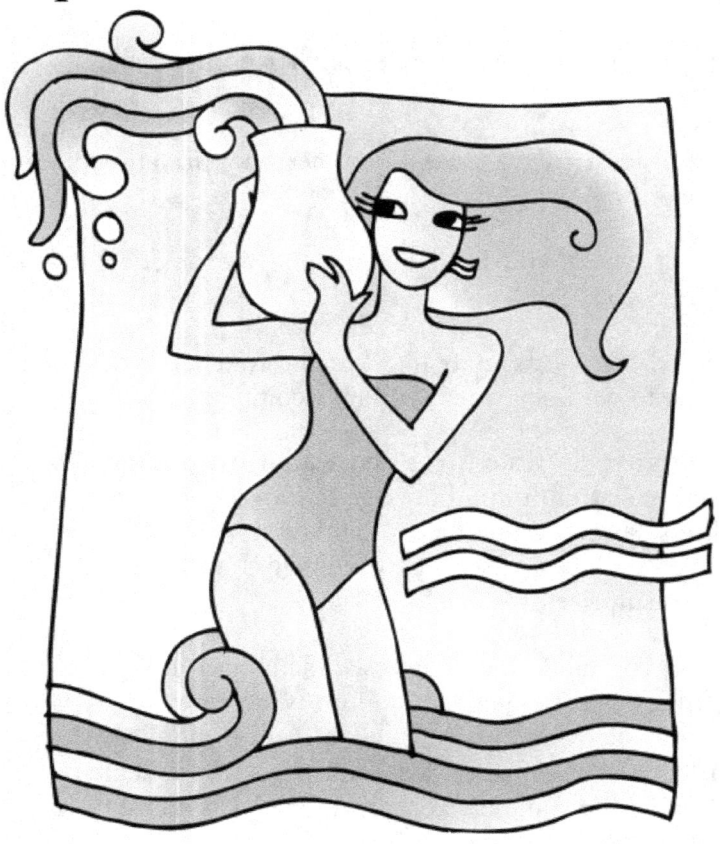

Fixed, Air, Masculine

Ruling planet: Saturn

Symbol: The Water Bearer

Diet Rating: 7/10

You are rebellious, unconventional and independent with a little kooky thrown in for good measure - right?

Aquarians march to the beat of their own drum, but it is a Saturn drum so there is an amount of credibility and determination that comes with your eccentricity.

Of course you will read an astrology book to help you lose weight. Why would anyone find that strange? Yes. I agree, but many people would think that we are both crazy and maybe we are a little – but it's the people who think outside the box that make the world so much more interesting.

So weight loss for you is connected to friends and ideas and just about anything that you can think of – because you are always thinking. And you know a lot – and sometimes it can be hard to tell you that you may not be right.

That's because you are stubborn and think that you know everything there is to know about everything. And maybe you do but here you are. Consulting an astrology book to help you lose weight – and you came to the right place!

I know you quite well and I believe we can come up with a superior plan that will have just the right elements to help you with your journey.

Aquarius is not really known for eating a whole lot of food. Sometimes you may just forget because you are thinking about something else that is far more important. Like your fellow Saturn-ruled sign – Capricorn – you have a lot of similar traits but it's just that you live in the world of ideas and concepts and they live in the earthy world of practicality. So they probably didn't buy the book anyway!

You could also be one of those people who has always been thin, eating whatever you like and then suddenly, one day in your thirties you think – what's with the weight gain? How did this happen?

If your metabolism has caught up with you it could be baby weight, hormone changes or simply a change of lifestyle – you gained or lost a partner or you moved countries for work and you haven't had time to establish a new routine.

Aquarius would also like to do everything with friends. While Capricorn can go it alone, you guys really don't like to because who else can you share your future oriented view of the world with if not your friends?

This is pretty easy – cut back, have a plan and stick to it. But whatever you do, make sure it's not boring! Boredom will have you screaming for the door. If something has left you off kilter in your life, then you need to find out what it is and make sure you get to the root of the problem.

Is it your circulation? Fluid retention in the ankles will show you that perhaps its time to dust off the walking shoes – no not those space boots you love so much – just the ordinary everyday sneakers, with colour and sparkles and you own individual style even when you are at the gym shoes.

What Aquarius needs for success:

Set a reasonable achievable goal with a *deadline* (you love deadlines)

Be practical about your time – you will probably go to the gym if this is part of your plan.

Rather than cut out food groups, reduce your portions (Saturn is all about less so this should be easy). Try new dishes,

Japanese or Thai food that has lots of fresh vegetables and seaweed and all kinds of strange food. You know you love it.

Count calories, lower your sugar intake, smaller portions and consistency are your goals.

Weigh yourself at least once a week – you need confirmation that things are working.

Learn by doing – you love trial and error and the practical experience it gives you.

Celebrity Aquarius such as Jennifer Aniston - who ate the same salad for 10 years while on Friends - routine, routine, build it in!! Paris Hilton and Ellen and

Oprah…OK so I could write a whole astrology book about Oprah. She is unique, different and exceptional in everything she does and her one issue that people know all about it weight. But this can be attributed to her Birthday Chart and her other two key points – Moon sign is Sagittarius and her Ascendant is Sagittarius. So with 2 Sagittarius and one Aquarius she would flip flop between the two.

Pisces

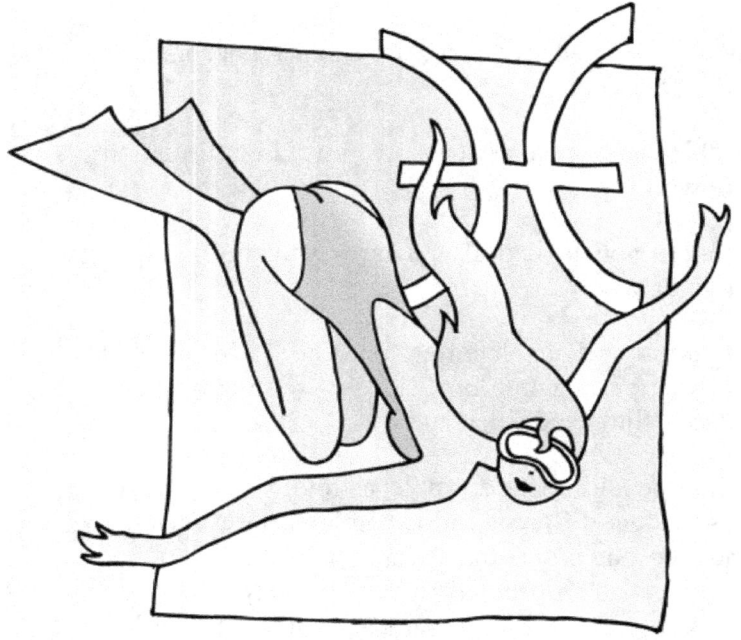

Mutable, Water, Feminine

Ruling Planet: Jupiter (No you are not ruled by Neptune!)

Symbol: The Fish

Diet Rating: 4/10

Pisces is a bit of a slippery fish. You may appear one way to some people and entirely another to others.

That's the duality of your sign, which is ruled by Jupiter (the biggest planet) Usually, Pisces is told how wonderful it is - a great sign – unlike those Scorpios with the sting in its tail or the two-faced Gemini hey!

Words like compassionate, kindness, creativity and imagination abound. But the other side of this sign is that these characteristics can easily lead to deception, being unrealistic or fanciful. You would love to live in a fantasy world and be completely irresponsible and sometimes you do!

Pisces is a mystery. Just when you think you get a handle on things you start questioning: What am I doing? Where am I? – Who am I? You can be a little dazed and confused yourself about who you are and what you believe. It's not that you mean to be like that, but sometimes you really do believe in your own publicity.

It can be very easy for you to create a fantasy world around you sometimes one of wishful thinking! You want the world to be a kind place where everyone is nice to one another. And you can be a little too easygoing

So now we are clear that I'm not letting you off the hook that easily (bad pun for the fish I know) the difficulty for anyone with strong Pisces energy is that you are able to twist and turn so easily and blame everyone else for your situation. You can't see yourself clearly and in many cases this leads to weight gain because you have a warped sense of what you look like in reality.

Have you ever looked at a photo and thought – is that really me? Do I look like that?

That's the kind of reality check Pisces needs to say – OK it really is time to do something about this.

Pisces is the most likely sign to mindlessly eat a whole a whole packet of biscuits while they are dreaming or thinking about something.

Willpower is not your strong suit is it?? While you do have some great qualities, being able to stick to things for a long period of time unless it is a fantasy, is not really how you operate – unless of course, your Birthday Chart has other factors.

Fantasy, dreams, movies are all big for Pisces. You can sense things that other signs cannot. Your intuition is strong. You can also hit the escape button and disappear – down a hole which is often linked to alcohol or drugs or some other escape from reality as it just *feels* better when you are dreaming.

What Pisces needs for success:

A reality check – try to be tough on yourself.

A plan that you can stick to easily – you tend to go for quick results rather than consistent over time. But if you did consistent over time it would be a lot easier!!

A vision of how you want to look and why you are doing this.

As a water sign water sports may be a good option

Pressure of any kind will make you fold – you need gentle reassurance from those around you.

Set small goals rather than one big goal. Break it down to smaller, manageable chunks.

You may not love exercise but usually love swimming or anything associated with water – like water skiing, surfing, aqua aerobics, standup paddle boarding etc

Try This:

You need to dream the dream, see the dream and then live it.

Try creative visualization – do a meditation where you can imagine your new self and lock that image in.

We need to start your program on a strong Saturn influence so that you stick to it!

Water retention may also be an issue – so try and reduce your salt intake and avoid or cut back on alcohol as it will be dehydrating.

Put a photo on your fridge that inspires you – it could be an old one of you or someone you admire

Exercise: Swimming! Anything you do either in or by the water will be of benefit. Also any time spent in the outdoors will be beneficial – they love nature. Dancing and other movement that includes music would also help you. Plug in your headphones and walk to your favourite music.

Make sure you have great shoes that fit well – your weakness is your feet so taking care of them is important.

Chapter 8 – Choosing the Program for your Horoscope Sign

Throughout the world there are so many programs, diets, pills and potions that promise you they will work. Sometimes and for some people they do.

For example, if you are a young fit person, then quite possibly an army style boot-camp 6-week program will adequately assist you and you can exercise yourself in to the ground and punish your poor body in to submission.

If you are over 50 and hoping to lose a few pounds, such strenuous exercise could be detrimental to your health.

I just did a quick Google search to locate the many options. They tend to fall in to a few categories:

Diet instructions and consultation in a group - organizations such as Weight Watchers

Food delivered – Lite n Easy (Australia) NutriFit (LA) Diet Chef (London)

Food provided and consultation – companies such as Jenny Craig

Shakes and meal replacements – products like Quick Trim, Herbalife, Celebrity Slim

Gyms and exercise – local groups and clubs

Self Reliant – menu plans, online, apps, etc

Aries – Top Picks - 6 2 and 5

Taurus – Top Picks – 2, 3 and 1

Gemini – Top Picks – 2,3 and 4

Cancer – Top Picks -2,3 and 1

Leo – Top picks - 6, 2 and 3

Virgo – Top Picks - 6, 5 and 3

Libra – Top Picks - 1, 3 and 2

Scorpio – Top Picks - 5, 6 and 3

Sagittarius – Top Picks - 3, 2 and 1

Capricorn – Top Picks - 6 4 and 1

Aquarius – Top Picks - 1, 6 and 4

Pisces – Top Picks 3, 2 and 1

I am not a nutritionist

I am not a qualified nutritionist so I can only be guided with my own experience and reading information that is available to everyone online.

As an astrologer however, I can give you some insight to your personality and how you can look at food, exercise and the different programs available to see if they resonate with you!

Here's what most people understand about weight loss:

Less food eaten + more exercise or movement = weight loss.

But if we break this down for the horoscope signs it is easy to see how differently we all manage to achieve this (or not!).

Reduce your calorie intake and move more

This seems like an easy step. But for some people they are not even aware of how many calories they eat in one day. I had no idea when I was young and the main thing I was getting wrong was portion control.

The size of your meal is very important. Some people with lots of will power can simply cut their meals in half.

So let's go through the signs to see if we can work out what will help you with reducing your calorie intake.

Fire signs – Aries, Leo, Sagittarius

Impatient and always on the move, the path of overeating for you seems to involve grabbing food and takeaway because you have no time for preparing meals and going grocery shopping.

The key here is to choose something that sets out a plan for you and means you have access to healthy alternatives if you are travelling or have lots of meetings each day and then come home and crash so you order take away.

Portion control for you will mean organization and substitutes. Shakes, juices and snacks like nuts and yoghurt could be great.

You also need to pay attention when you eat so make sure you put some time aside for your meals. Plan a list on the weekend and have your meals organized.

Home delivery services of fresh meals and snacks will really help you avoid high calorie takeaways.

Portion control is also important – try to weigh things if you can or just realize that standard meals have become so huge that if you cut them in half you probably have about the right amount of calories.

Fire signs have so much flair that they rarely look at the details – but it's the details with food that may surprise you. Try and keep a diary of what you eat for a week and look at where you can cut back (be very honest with yourself!)

Exercise and Movement:

Fire signs are all about movement. You love to run around and be active. Well most of you (check your other astro points – Moon and Ascendant – and read the description here for those signs too).

Fire signs usually like to sweat – Leo is naturally hot anyway (you guys are ruled by the sun)

Partying and socializing are also your big thing – you love to dance and be with others – so groups where you are also enjoying some movement are great for you.

Remember not to indulge too much in alcohol as this will add to your waistline and you may find that just reducing your drinking if you are a big partygoer will help.

Try one alcoholic beverage and then one soda or mineral water. Avoid sugary mixers with your drink – so try Vodka and soda with fresh lime rather than Vodka and cranberry juice.

Earth signs - Taurus, Virgo and Capricorn

Eating less for you may seem difficult. You love food – and it must be great quality. Taurus usually loves high fat, comfort food and you like snakes such as potato chips, crunchy salty and sweets, chocolate etc. So here are my top tips for you.

Do not cut out whole food groups like Carbs – that is just too drastic and even with the willpower you have (your famous stubbornness – who me?) yes even you will have trouble doing this for long periods of time.

For you, it is important that you have access to all the treats you love – try something that offers you substitutes for that taste.

The pleasure of the senses is Taurus big issue – yet if you cut your meals in half – you would probably be OK. One trick I heard was to use a small plate – that way it looks like more. Also fill up on salad, vegetables and other low calorie options then you will feel fuller.

Remember – if you are hungry that means you are losing weight. For some Taurus this is difficult to remember – so apples, nuts and other vegetable snacks bulk up on – and cut down on the high fat.

Another trick for your sign is to eat really well for most of the time and have treats for 20% of the time. This type of program will work better for you in the maintenance phase as it is difficult to get the weight of with this method.

Exercise and Movement

Earth signs need to walk on the earth! Take your shoes off and walk in the grass like Richard Gere did in that scene from the movie Pretty Woman! Connecting your bare feet to the earth will help you connect with the natural pulse of the planet.

Taurus you need to walk. Capricorn, you guys love to climb. Virgo you guys need to work on your nerves and sleep.

At the very least, if you can work towards doing these things this will help you with your weight loss.

All signs will benefit from lower alcohol intake. The pleasures of eating and drinking are a big one for our earthly existence.

Remember to look after your body and don't push it too much. So low impact may be better for you – no need to pump weights – just walking will help you and make it an easy walk so that you can do small increments each day.

So if you are not very sporty, for the first day just walk for 20 minutes – that's just 10 minutes in one direction and then turning around and walking back. After you feel you have built up some steam – go to 30 minutes and before you know it you will want to walk for an hour.

Set this in to your schedule – because earth signs are practical. You like to know what is happening each day and if you just build it in to your daily routine you will barely notice as the weight drops off!

Air signs – Gemini, Libra and Aquarius

Nervous energy is the problem of the Twins – if you are stressed you will probably eat more and turn to those foods you love that are comforting.

To reduce your food intake you need to up the foods that help your nervous system – nuts, (cashews and macadamia nuts) fresh fruits and vegetables like berries, asparagus, avocado and drinks without caffeine such as chamomile and green tea.

The other thing about nerves is that it will make you anxious about your life in general which means planning goes out the window and you are left eating lots of takeaway food.

Planning is your friend and this will also help to relieve your stress.

The third thing for a Mercury ruled sign is socializing – your party life means that you love a drink and when you are drinking too much you may forget about your portion controls and eat too much food.

One of the best tips for parties is to make sure you don't go on an empty stomach.

Eat some yoghurt and nuts before you leave or a slice of wholemeal toast with some avocado so you don't feel like eating all the finger food!

Also keep a watch on the calories in your drinks. A glass of wine, vodka and soda with a slice of lime or lemon, or a glass of champagne are all better choices than beer or sweet, creamy cocktails that are loaded with calories.

Exercise and Movement

You are an air sign so getting out in the fresh air is good for you! Breathing deeply will help you immensely – things like yoga are perfect for you. You also love being social and fashionable – so going to a dance class, gym or other meeting place may also appeal to you.

Solitary pursuits are not usually your thing but if you give them a chance it could be very good for you to go for a long walk by yourself. This will calm your mind – and we are trying to release stress that is based on your thinking overload!

Another word of warning for Air signs – it is not a great idea to go to the gym before you go to bed. Your heart and mind will be racing and this could impact on your sleep. You need at least 8 hours sleep a night as your nervous system needs time to recuperate.

Reading is a great way for you to wind down. Do not have television sets or your mobile/cell phone in your bedroom – if you do cover them up with a blanket. Research from Harvard and University of Toronto (Harvard Health Publications – www.health.harvard.edu) found that light in the blue spectrum acts on our bodies by suppressing natural melatonin so keep it out of your bedroom or you may have problems getting drowsy and dosing off to sleep

Water Signs – Cancer, Scorpio and Pisces

For the water signs it's important to get a grip on your emotional eating. As the most sensitive signs in the zodiac you really feel things very strongly which means that even the anticipation of a fight or argument will have you reaching for the biscuit tin (cookie jar!).

Keeping calm and having your relationships with family, friends and co-workers on an even keel will be your best bet for weight loss.

Walking in nature, going for a swim in the ocean or having an animal you can care for are all ways that will help you channel your feelings.

Sweetness is your weakness! I know you love chocolate – nearly everyone does but for you it's like taking a chill pill! My best tip for you is to learn to love dark chocolate.

Dark chocolate has less sugar and fat than milk chocolate and if you get a good brand (like a Swiss or European chocolate) just a few small pieces usually satisfies even the worst sweet tooth! I agree it is bitter and I was reluctant to try it, but give it a go.

If you have a small piece with a cup of herbal tea at night it may help you with the night munchies. If ice-cream is another weakness go for a frozen yogurt (but make sure you check the sugar and calories).

Don't have sweet foods in the house. If you have children – that's no excuse! Fruit and healthy alternatives are great for them too. If it's not in the house then you are less likely to reach for it.

The same goes for wine or alcohol – you can have one small glass a day but not if you have desert after dinner.

Exercise and Movement

Water sports and swimming are wonderful ways for you to exercise. Hiking and walking in nature is also a great way for you to help calming yourself and get on that even keel.

I think meditation and listening to music is also a great way to relax and with your strong imagination creative visualization is also a tool that works.

Basically you need to have rewards that are not food – so think about other ways you can reward yourself – a pedicure, a massage, watching a movie, calling a friend. Think of the things you love to do and when the emotional eating feeling starts to rise – occupy yourself.

All kinds of crafts like knitting, quilting and sewing are also great – because water signs are also very creative. Think of the time you can spend making things that will keep you occupied and away from the refrigerator!

Basics for every sign

Reduce your calorie intake by reducing the size of your meals

Have three healthy snacks per day in between meals

Move more and build it in to your routine

Get more sleep – at least 8 hours and (no TV or electronics in the bedroom)

Get any junk food out of the house before you start

Don't go for trendy or fashionable diets – these fads come and go. We are looking for something that will help you long term

Aim for a balanced diet – fruit and vegetables, whole grains, lean protein and a few treats sprinkled throughout the week will be good.

Cut down on sugar

Nuts like cashews, almonds and walnuts are great for reducing hunger

Remember to include drinks – reduce sugary drinks and alcohol

Drink plenty of water!

If you are serious – this will be something you can do. And with the magic intention it will be easier to stick to than in the past.

Check out my website – www.starsandthecity.com for some menu ideas and eating plans for the week.

Chapter 9 - Now for the Magic!

If you start your diet on a Monday you are practically doomed from the start. How many people start a diet on a Monday? Here's why it's not a good idea:

The days of the week are each ruled by a particular heavenly body:

Monday – Moon

Tuesday – Mars

Wednesday – Mercury

Thursday – Jupiter

Friday – Venus

Saturday – Saturn

Sunday – Sun

The sign of the Moon in your Birthday Chart explains your emotions. As the Moon is the fastest moving body listed above, it changes signs very quickly. It is too *changeable* for you to anchor your diet.

Technically I suppose you could start on a Monday and have success (particularly if the moon was in a stable sign) but we are aiming for less of a struggle and for that Saturn is your guy.

Saturn rules structure, determination, achievement, solid foundations, longevity and steadfastness. For commencing a diet regime this is what we need – right?

We might use Tuesday Friday or Sunday as alternatives but forget about Monday, and Wednesday.

Thursday is ruled by Jupiter that is the biggest planet and has a tendency to just make things bigger. Enough said.

Phases of the Moon

The other really important element of choosing a time and date for your start time is the phase of the moon.

We will do a little Primary School science when we get to that section, but for the moment we need to know that when the moon is at its New Moon phase growing to become a full moon this is called a Waxing Moon. This is when you plant seeds and hope they will grow. Not what we want - right?

The phase we are looking for is the phase after the Full Moon until the next New Moon which is called the Waning Moon. A waning moon is perfect for us. As the moon shrinks in size we hope to shrink with it.

How do we know what phase the moon is in? It's pretty easy to work out and there are many places online that will tell you. There are even apps you can download to give you the phases of the moon.

My website www.starsandthecity.com.au will update the phases of the Moon and each month I will list the best days to commence your diet.

So don't worry – I will make sure you know the perfect time to commence your Weight Loss Lunar Magic.

The History of Magic and Ceremony

The world really is a much more magical place that we currently give it credit. We are at the very end of a cycle that is based on earth signs (reality, things I can touch and feel, money, land etc).

However, as humans our bodies are so much more than the physical. You have heard the saying mind over matter and scientists use that to dissuade people from things. For example if people take a pill in a scientific study - like an Aspirin and they actually get results they say: "Oh that's just the placebo effect"

So without going into too much complicated scientific material in this book – there are plenty of others out there for you to read if you want more information – but the overall understanding many of us now have about our bodies is that they are unbelievably complex and our minds are like the central control centre.

Other civilizations have known this for thousands of years. Indigenous cultures understand that there are many dimensions to who we are and that the body is just the vessel for the soul. This is how shamanic work happens and people can be "magically" cured.

What we are about to embark on is simple Moon magic. It involves an understanding that the cycle of the moon has a beginning, middle and end.

And for women this is really important. As the moon representative of the feminine it rules out cycles. We are in a world that is predominantly masculine or Sun oriented and here is how the astrology explains this.

The western world runs on the Gregorian calendar which has 12 months in a year right? And there is this weird issue with February where we change the number of days in a leap year – (this allows us to catch up with the Sun's 365 and a quarter day cycle.

But go and get your calculator. Type in 365 (for the days of the year) and then divide this by 28) and you will get an incredible answer: 13.

Really this is amazing. There are 13 cycles of the moon within the year and we struggle and add days here and there to certain months and worry every four years about extra days – when it could be simple – just give us 13 months and we can then understand our feminine cycle better than we currently do given the calendar we use.

It is also believed that this is where the superstition about the number 13 originates as the foundation of our masculine based society is actually fearful of women and our ability to give birth!

Astrologically, the year is divided into four seasons and these are based around the Sun's apparent movement in the sky. The Solstices and Equinoxes divide the year into – summer, autumn, winter and spring.

The Equinoxes and Solstices

This is when the Sun crosses the Tropic of Capricorn (Northern Hemisphere Winter Solstice and the Southern Hemisphere experiences Summer Solstice) and occurs around the time of 21 December. (We say around this date because it can change dates due to the reasons I have already outlined. But for our simple purposes I will just say around these dates!)

When the Sun crosses the Tropic of Cancer this marks the Northern Hemisphere Summer Solstice and Southern Hemisphere Winter Solstice and occurs around 21 June.

An equinox occurs when the Sun crosses the equator, which occurs twice during the year:

Around 21 March – Equinox – spring for the Northern Hemisphere and autumn or fall for the Southern Hemisphere.

Around 21 September – Equinox – autumn for the Northern Hemisphere and spring for the Southern Hemisphere.

In astrological terms this is as follows:

Around 21 March – Sun moves in to the sign of Aries to mark the beginning of the year.

Around 21 June – Sun moves in to the sign of Cancer

Around 21 September – Sun moves in to the sign of Libra

Around 21 December – Sun moves in to the sign of Capricorn.

We call this the cardinal ingress because the sun moves in to the cardinal signs of Aries, Cancer, Libra and Capricorn.

Moon Cycle

The Moon moves through each sign of the zodiac each 28-29 day period. This changes every year and most astrologers will have a list of the new moon and full moon cycles for the year on their web site.

You can find it on my site – www.starsandthecity.com

Once in the yearly cycle there will be a new moon in each sign and a full moon in each sign.

New Moon

At the new moon the sky is dark and you cannot see the moon. It is when the Sun and the Moon are together in the sky – in the same astrological sign.

This phase is a time of beginnings. It is a time for planting seeds and starting any project that you want to grow! It is always good to start something when the moon is in a fertile sign and you can be sure that it will be strong.

During the phase from the New Moon to the full moon we are going from not being able to see it – to full illumination. This is called the waxing phase and is a time for things getting bigger! Not a good time for starting a diet. So we will be sure not to start our program during this phase.

I would also like to reiterate that astrologers take in to account so many variables that it is better - if at all possible – have an astrologer look at your individual chart you will get a stronger result.

I will keep an up-to-date list on my website and endeavor to keep some information on the Stars and the City Facebook page. This will also be a place where we can talk about the Moon and what phase and sign it is in, so that you can get current information to help you.

Full Moon

At the full moon the moon is illuminated – as it is seen from our place on earth. It is the time when the Sun and the Moon are opposite each other. This is a time when we can fully see what is happening.

The phase where the moon goes from full to new is called the waning phase. This is a time when it is no good to plant things or start anything new. It is a time of reaping what you have sown, releasing, pulling out weeds and getting ready for the new cycle ahead.

As we want to go from full to less full – this is the best time for starting a diet as we are losing what we no longer need.

So the phase of the moon will help you and I will list the dates and times on my website and social media so that you can ask questions and get some help to learn when it is the best time to start your diet program.

Chapter 10 – Ready for the Weight Loss Ceremony

Does the thought of magic mean witchcraft and scary things to you? And what is a witch today?

This is quite a difficult question to answer and possibly there is no correct answer. You may like to think of witches as ugly old crones with warts on their nose and riding a broomstick – and this is how many people still dress during Halloween!

But others may see witches like Samantha in Bewitched, or any of the beautiful women in Charmed and quite possibly there are many of you who associate magic and witchcraft with the Harry Potter series of books and think of both men and women as creating magic – that is not about any "witchiness" at all!

There is no doubt that religions give witchcraft a bad name and I think it means so many different things to different people that I can only give you my own personal view and offer you some great reading material if you want to explore this area more fully!

Magic is divided into a number of areas that include ceremonial magic and all kinds of horrible things like curses and people trying to gain control over other people or events.

My idea of magic is that it is the natural kind of magic – where you try to find synchronicity in your surroundings and you ask God or your angels, guides, or even ascended masters to assist you with your ceremony.

Ceremony is important because it provides a focus and intention for your magic. There are lots of tools available that can help you, like crystals and candles and really all these are designed to do is focus your thoughts and energy.

Then there is you! And you are a very important part of the equation, as is your history, culture and belief system. It doesn't matter what religion you are, there are many people who still understand the old ways of the culture and today this is found in superstitions and ways in which we try to make sense of customs.

So for my cultural roots I feel safe in the Celtic roots of my family and the ancient civilizations such as Egypt which I have a natural curiosity. I love going to see the Egyptian section of the Metropolitan Museum in New York and have spent hours there just looking at the artifacts and I find it endlessly fascinating.

So follow your intuition on this one. What interests you about past civilizations? Which family members do you associate with most strongly?

I love the idea of fairies and elves, leprechauns and garden spirits that can help you – it just seems that if you look for it there is magic everywhere! From finding a white feather if you are thinking of a deceased loved one, to simple things like you are thinking of a friend and they suddenly call you. There is so much more to the world than we currently admit in our education systems and media, but that does not stop many of us from believing.

Natural magic is what I believe in and it is a form of white magic that uses nature to assist you and help you with a desired outcome. If you then write down your desire and send it out to the universe, you will be surprised how this can help you in so many ways – not just with weight loss!

So here are my simple steps that have been pulled together like the Gemini magpie I truly am and I would like to acknowledge just some of the books and authors who have helped me on this magical journey so I have listed some authors and books at the back for you to explore.

The list goes on and on but this is a great starting point if you want to learn a little more. Many people who are involved in magic also want to learn about astrology because it is the foundation of so much of this information.

I do understand that magic can be far more complicated and very dangerous if you are dabbling in an area that you don't fully understand. So stay in the shallow pool with your floating devises attached at all times!

Never, Ever, EVER – try to do magic that is aimed at a particular person or getting an outcome that involves changing the freewill of someone else.

This will backfire on you badly – even if you think what I'm talking about is just a bit of a laugh or it is rubbish – don't do it.

What we are doing involves YOUR freewill which involves changing your perception and changing your habits. It is never about someone else. After all, the only person that needs to change in changing your body is you!

Clearing Yourself

Chances are that if this is the first book you have picked up that even has anything to do with magic, and you have no idea that you are in possession of a fabulous body! You really are!

It can do so many amazing things and we never give it credit but perhaps it's about time to think of your body as a wonderful temple that you need to look after for your experience on this planet to be a happy, joyous experience!

Always remember – you are a beautiful soul who has come to this time and place on this planet to learn new things, to enjoy life and once you have mastered this – to help others.

Your body is a reflection of your ability to process so many things that are not food related.

It is possible that old emotions are stuck in your body and this is causing you problems. Thoughts and any ideas or beliefs that are stuck in your mental body can also be causing you to hold on to weight.

This is why we need to clear you first. Think about this for a little while:

Am I upset with someone and unable to tell them what I think?

Is there something in my past that happened that makes me scared just to think about it?

Is there an incident, something that happened to you or something that was said that has made you feel bad?

If you have been overweight for some time – when was the first time you remember being overweight – was there something that happened with your parents or with your family that made you feel different or not good about yourself?

If you are nodding to any of these questions chances are that you are holding on to something that could have an impact on your ability to move forward and be the ideal weight you would like to be.

This could have happened a long time ago and you don't realize the impact it has had on you.

I have worked with many healers over the years and I'm sure you can find someone near you who can help you with this – if it is something you think you need to explore further than what I am about to outline here.

Whenever I need someone I just put it out there to the universe that I need someone to help me with an issue and usually a friend or someone I know will give me the name of a person who has helped them in a similar way.

It never ceases to amaze me how the universe works and how I always find the perfect practitioner to assist me! You can do this too – just think about it or write it down and you will find someone.

Some of the people who may be able to help include natural or holistic healers such as:

Life counseling or coaching, hypnotherapy, Reiki, Energy healing, Flower Essence Therapists, NLP practitioners, kinesiology, Yoga, Meditation or Past Life Regression.

It is better to be guided or to have someone recommend any of the above practitioners. In the end, you need to see someone who is reputable and can really help you.

I must admit as I wrote this list I can tick the box of many of these, but remember it is your journey and you need to find someone with whom you feel comfortable.

These people address the whole person – physical, mental, emotional and spiritual wellbeing is considered in the treatment programs they offer. They will often be people who encourage their patients to take responsibility for their own health as they assist you with helping to find the root cause of an issue.

If you are a person who is taking lots of medication, it may be a good idea to talk to your own doctor and get some ideas from them as to how you can work to resolve any emotional issues.

How do I clear myself?

Yoga and meditation are great ways to clear yourself and your own energy field. They are both simple and cheap and you can find free videos on YouTube now to help you to calm yourself or release any emotions you have been holding on to.

I will put some videos up on my own channel soon – so check out www.starsandthecity.com for links to the videos.

Flower essence drops are also great for helping your physical body release old emotions. You can usually find these at a health food store or I can highly recommend that you find a practitioner who will mix your own special bottle.

Burning essential oils is another way of helping to calm and reduce stress. Oils such as Lavender are great and can be used in the bath too.

One of the best ways I find to relax before I do any energy work is to have a bath, put the oils in with the bubbles and play chakra clearing music.

Or if you are feeling more energetic, a walk or run along a beach or in nature will help to clear your energy. Just putting your bare feet on the grass and feeling the sun on your body is also a wonderful way to clear your energy field. Try it the next sunny day!

Try This:

Run a bath with some salt (can be bath salts or just ordinary table salt)

Drop essential oils associated with your sign in to the bath.

Light a candle

Play some music and relax while you say

"I release all my stress in to the bath water"

"I feel good about myself"

Thank you universe for cleansing my aura"

Call in Archangel Raphael to help heal your body.

When you get out - Put some more oil on your body and look in the mirror and smile. Be Happy – you are a beautiful Goddess (or God)

Clearing Your Space

While it's important to try and keep your energy field clear while you are losing weight – your home is also important. The best way to keep your home clear is to smudge it.

Smudging is just simply burning something that will smoke up and as the smoke fills the air you walk around asking the universe to bless your space and release it. If you are new to this ask an Archangel such as Metatron or Michael to help you.

You can get dried sage online, put it in a fireproof dish and light it.

While it's burning make sure it is in a safe place and that you don't drop any cinders or set anything on fire - please!

When you have finished – open all the doors and windows for a few minutes and let it flow out.

Make sure you extinguish the sage fully. The best way to do this is stave it of oxygen – so put a lid on the dish and it will stop burning.

There are lots of sprays you can use to clear your space – some are available online or you may be able to get one in a New Age or health food store. Common ones include sage, citronella, lavender and frankincense.

Selecting your Day

To find the best day for you we need to look at the Moon Cycle and make sure it is just after the full Moon. All these dates will be posted on my website or in social media – Facebook etc.

We need a day that will help you stick to your plan and I have always found that Saturday is a great day – things will stick alright and you will be able to continue your diet as long as necessary.

People often ask me does it have to be Saturday – I have a party or that my social time. So of course there are other days during the cycle and they can include:

Friday – day of Venus – if you are strong Taurus or Libran energy

Tuesday – day of Mars – if you are strong in Aries or Scorpio energy

The other days are a bit too changeable for my liking. I will also look at the months ahead and give you dates – because sometimes you need a few weeks to get organized. We will also look at the sign the Moon will be in and any aspects that are being made to the Moon.

Of course it is always better if you get an individual reading and I can help you with this. I have a special rate for looking at your chart and giving you your three power points – Sun, Moon and ascendant sign.

Sometimes you may not know your birth time so I can have a look at other planets and houses and give you some insight. I can also suggest the best days for you to start. So don't worry if you find this all a little confusing – there is help available thanks to social media and email.

Starting your diet on that day means waking up and that is the day you change your food and exercise habits.

To do your ceremony – you can do this the day or night before.

For example – I always like to do the ceremony on the day of Venus as this is a great day for all things feminine. I then wake up on Saturday and start my diet.

Other days that would work well would be to do the ceremony on a Monday – the day of the Moon and this is lunar magic! Then you would wake up on the Tuesday and start – with is the day of Mars and a great day for determination and getting things done.

Selecting your magic items

We need to keep this part very simple. The nature of magic is that it works with the four elements – Fire Earth Air and Water (in that order) and the four directions North South West and East.

To satisfy the four elements you need something from each of these for your magic:

Fire – Candle (best to use white candles here)

Earth – A crystal (a quartz or red/orange stone) paper, pen

Air – incense, essential oils like cinnamon or ginger spray or rub

Water – a cup or glass of water (filtered is good if you don't have that then cooled boiled water)

Now you can choose any of these you like – but I like white, red or pink candles, amethyst or clear quartz crystals, and an essential oil that resonates with your sign. Lavender and frankincense seems to work well for just about everything. Put the water in a red cup or clear glass.

But the best part of this ceremony is that it is yours and you get to choose. The other very important thing is that you can call on your guides, Jesus, Angels or just about anyone else you pray to or ask for help and guidance to help you with your ceremony.

In Christian cultures Angels and Jesus are popular. But in other cultures, Buddah or another guide may be more appropriate. The Hindus for example will have many Gods and Goddesses they can call on and will use the most appropriate for this ceremony and for breaking down blockages Ganesh would be wonderful to call on and ask for assistance.

Below is another list that may help you and you can just choose a name that feels right for you.

Your guides,

Angels – Archangel Michael and Raphael, Apollo,

Jesus or Mary

Hindu God Ganesh is a great remover of obstacles.

A departed loved one who you have a special relationship may also be able to help you (like your nana or other family members)

Think about this list for a few days before and ask the guide who feels most appropriate to help you with your ceremony and your weight loss journey.

Ready for Ceremony
Checklist:

Know your date and time –

I will also post some times for you as there are certain magic hours (called planetary hours) that can also help, but once again – go with what feels right and a time you know you can be alone.

I know people who have families and children who have either waited until everyone is in bed and done this while they are alone or locked themselves in a bedroom and asked their partner not to disturb them.

So just go with whatever works best for you!

Gather all your tools together.

Have everything including matches or a lighter assembled in the one place so that you are not running around during the ceremony.

I am currently putting together little parcels for you that I will have on my website. If you have purchased a package from the Stars and the City website you will have everything you need and then you just need to make sure you have the matches and the water.

Cleanse yourself and your space.

This can be as long as going through the bath and smudging exercises outlined above or as simple as having a sage spray that you spray above your head and in the area you want because you did the clearing a few days ago.

I would say that up to a week your space is good and with the other elements of this ceremony you should be fine. Go with how you feel.

Place all your items in front of you on the floor

(I'm guessing you don't have an altar but if you do then you can use that or a low table) it is better if you can sit on the floor for this – but I know some of you won't want to do this and that is OK. You can sit on a chair or stand. You just need these items within easy reach and they have to be in your circle area.

OK here we go!

Close your eyes and ground yourself. Imagine you are connected to the earth via little cords that grow out of the bottom of your spine.

Take a deep breath and imagine a circle of white lights around you – a circle that is big enough to fill the room.

Ask your guide for help – This can be as simple as: "I ask my guides and Jesus to please help me with this ceremony."

Light your candle.

Pick up your crystal and hold it in your hand (the one other than the one you write with.)

Spray your essential oil spray or have your incense or oil burning. You can also rub this oil on your hands.

Look in to the water and breathe deeply three times.

Then write down your intention. It could be something like this:

To the Universe, Dear God

Thank you for helping me in the coming weeks to lose _____ Kgs or lbs

I ask you to please help me release any addictions to XYZ (sugar, junk food or alcohol etc) and help me find great substitutes so that I don't even crave them.

I also ask for help with choosing more healthy food options like fresh fruit and vegetables.

Please help me find interesting ways to incorporate them in my daily meals.

I would also like to be able to stick to my new eating and exercise plan easily and effortlessly so that I just do it without even thinking about it. It is EASY!

Thank you for your help and guidance and I know you will be with me every day assisting me to lose this weight.

Then sign your name and write the date.

Remember this is YOUR spell. So you can write and include whatever you want!

Then say this:

I call in the elements of fire, earth air and water to help me with my weight loss.

I call in Archangel Raphael (or other helper you have chosen) to assist me with this health issue so that I can lose weight easily and effortlessly.

Now read your note out loudly and strongly and feel the emotion when you say it (that is - say it like you *really* mean it, don't just read it – *feel* it).

Then say - So be it! (You can also say So be it mote or Amen or any other ending)

Wait a few moments and soak in what you have just asked for. Visualise yourself at your new weight and the new clothes you will buy or old jeans that you will fit in to.

Drink the water.

Then release the four elements:

I release the four elements – fire, earth, air and water

I release any guides, Archangels, helpers etc

Say this as you snuff out the candle (with a spoon or a lid but **don't blow it out**)

Take your crystal, and put it under your bed (or near your bed) with the paper and the note you wrote.

There you are – you did it! Now you have asked the universal energy field to help you and you have strongly and carefully identified the ways in which you need help and how much weight you want to lose. Congratulations on setting your Weight Loss lunar Magic spell.

What's next?

Now that you have done the magic forget about it. The key to magic is to have such a belief that it will work that you don't need to worry about it. This is what I call allowing it to happen.

Over the coming weeks you may want to keep a journal about how you feel and how the process of losing weight is happening.

Now that you have done your intention you can start your "diet" or new eating program the following day.

The day you start will be the date we have chosen.

For example if you are starting your diet on a Saturday or Tuesday or the waxing moon phase – you will do your intention ceremony either that day before you start or the night before.

Please join me on social media – Facebook and Twitter – www.StarsandtheCity.com – and I hope to post lots of videos on my YouTube channel that will help you learn more and may even answer some of the questions you have!

I would love to hear from you about your journey and your results.

I wish everyone the best and hope you have a wonderful time on your weight loss journey!

Lots of Love and Best Wishes for Amazing Success!

Julie Ann xxx

Chapter 11 – Common Questions and Answers

I know there will be lots of questions but please keep in mind that this is your spell and you can really do whatever you like!

But just in case I have put together some commonly asked questions. If you have any further questions I look forward to chatting to you on social media.

Does it have to be at the date and time you say?

Yes – it is better to do this intention ceremony on the date and time suggested as we are following the cycle of the moon and using the planets to go with us.

It's a bit like swimming against the tide rather than going with the flow and floating – it is much less of a struggle and that is the whole purpose of the ceremony.

What if I miss the time?

If you miss the time on the day you choose – there may be another good time over the coming weeks. Don't worry!

However if the moon becomes a new moon and it is at the waxing stage of its cycle, then you will have to wait two weeks until after the full moon.

That's OK. Sometimes the universe knows what it is doing and perhaps it is better for you to get more organized and start a little bit later than you thought.

Why is there no meal plan to follow?

We are all so different these days that if I put a meal plan here there would be lots of people writing to me saying - I'm vegetarian or I'm gluten free or I have an allergy to this food.

There are so many different plans available that you will have any number of choices. I have listed some of the ways you could make your choice based on your horoscope sign and your Birthday Chart.

It is much easier for you to find a diet program – for women that is 1200 calories per day and for men – 1800 calories per day that is aligned with your preferences.

If you read the astrology section and look at your sign for the Sun, Moon and Ascendant Signs you can also get some good ideas as to the style of diet that suits you.

What exercise should I do?

If you have read your horoscope signs for the Sun, Moon and Ascendant and you still don't know what the best exercise is for you – then walk! It is free, easy and low impact.

If you are snow bound or do not have a place to walk near you then either a treadmill or a low impact exercise DVD will be great.

But I have lost weigh many times with very little exercise – so it can be done.

Really it is about how much you are eating and your determination to keep going.

The longer you can go on any diet program and the slower your weight loss the safer it is for you and you are more likely to keep it up. This is because you are forming great new habits.

I don't know how to read my chart and find my astrology points

If you cannot work out your three key astrology points – Sun, Moon and Ascendant then there are a few ways you may be able to get help.

I have mini readings available just for this purpose and I will send you an email or a MP3 sound file that will give you your three points.

If you don't know what time you were born then your Sun and Ascendant signs will be considered the same.

What if all of my signs are the same?

It is possible to have the same Sun, Moon and Ascendant signs. If this is the case for you then it means you are a triple sign and the emphasis of that sign on your characteristics is very strong.

Make sure you read that sign carefully and be aware of your strengths and weaknesses.

If I haven't covered all your questions here – then please go to my website or social media – Facebook etc and ask a question. I will be happy to answer any questions you may have there.

What other books do you recommend that may help give you some more detail about magic?

Scott Cunningham (Earth Air Fire and Water is one of the best books on this type of magic)

Christopher Penczak - (bit more advanced but incredibly readable)

Gregg Braden (if you like a little more scientific info)

Doreen Virtue (Angels, Guides, she is just the best)

James Redfield (Celestine Prophecy – hard to go past if you are a beginner)

Deborah Gray and Fiona Horne - (two Australian witches who published some of the first books I read on magic).